HEART
SEIZURES

HEART SEIZURES

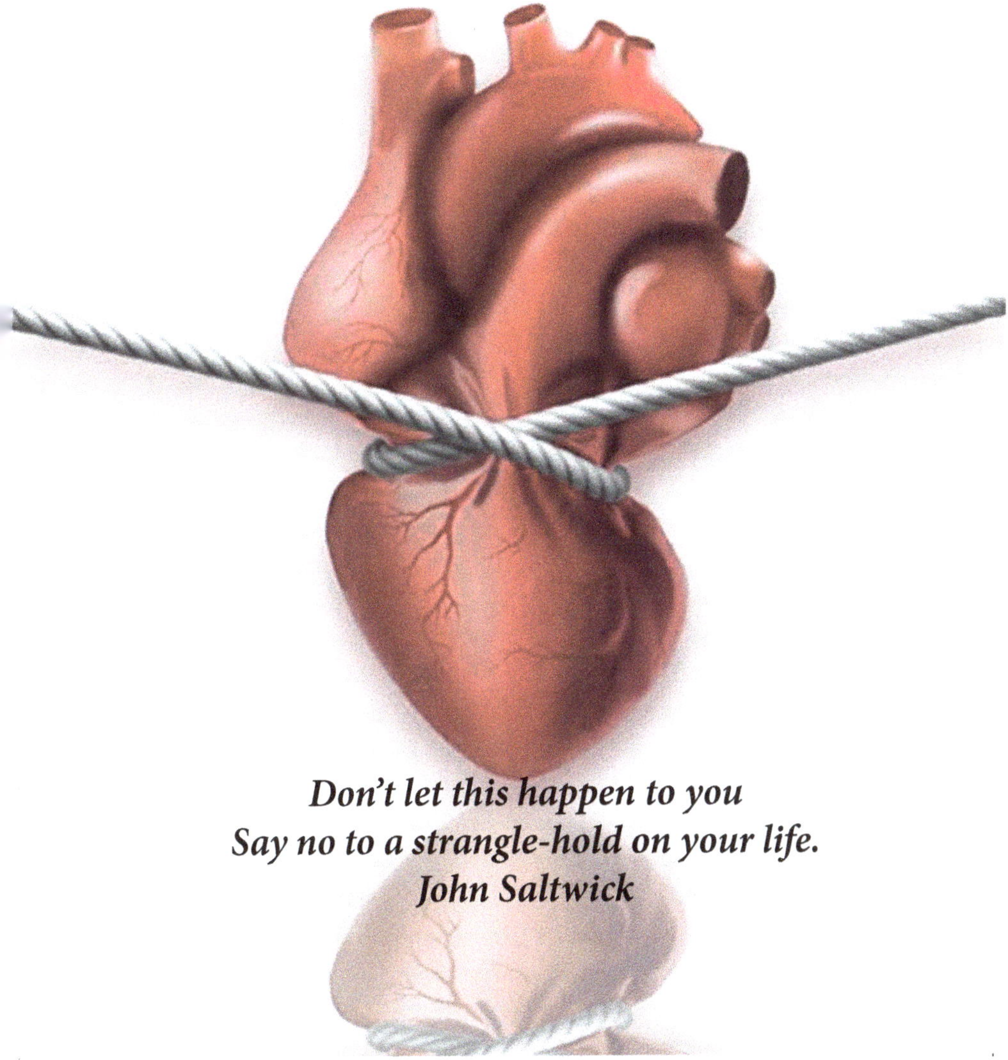

Don't let this happen to you
Say no to a strangle-hold on your life.
John Saltwick

CITI OF
BOOKS

CITIOFBOOKS, INC.
3736 Eubank NE Suite A1
Albuquerque, NM 87111-3579
www.citiofbooks.com
Hotline: 1 (877) 389-2759
Fax: 1 (505) 930-7244

Ordering Information:
Quantity sales. Special discounts are available on quantity purchases by corporations, associations, and others. For details, contact the publisher at the address above.

Printed in the United States of America.

ISBN-13:	Softcover	979-8-89391-403-0
	eBook	979-8-89391-404-7

Library of Congress Control Number: 2024921580

Table of Contents

Disclaimer

The intent of this book is to be a reference volume and chronology of one person's bout with and management of coronary artery disease (CAD) and not as a medical manual. The information laid out in this book is what the author learned over twenty years while defying the odds of living with coronary artery disease and is not a substitute for medical doctor intervention. Hopefully the information in this book will promote examination and thinking about the heart and heart attacks and help the reader to understand coronary artery disease and the treatment prescribed by his or her physician.

Mention in this book of specific organizations, associations, companies and authorities does not in any way imply endorsement of those organizations by the publisher and the author, nor does their mention herein imply in any way an endorsement by them of this book.

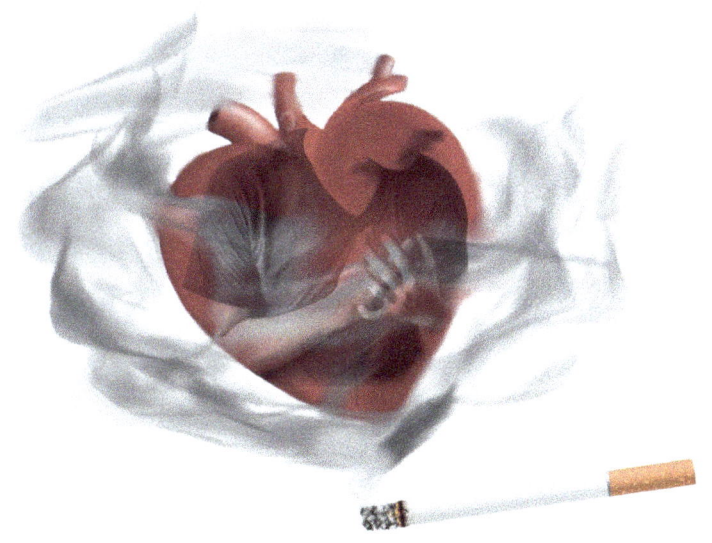

Chapter 1

Some years ago, with my morning cup of coffee in hand, I went up to my smoking lounge, an outdoor balcony where I could stand and marvel at the view of the Olympic mountains spread out before me and the ships traversing the broad expanse of Puget Sound. Every morning, I would stand there with my coffee and enjoy the first of roughly sixty plus cigarettes for the day. You got it, I smoked on average three packs a day; and occasionally as many as four. After about the fourth puff, I started feeling a tightness in my chest. It was like a heavy weight was pressing down on me. Having never felt it before, I wrote it off as heartburn. I figured it was from something I ate the night before or possibly I had made the coffee too strong. Grinding out my cigarette, I went down to my office, two floors below. To my dismay, the tightness in my chest persisted. It had not disappeared. Seated in my office, I tried to ignore any discomfort I felt and focused on what I had to do that day.

After about a half hour the tightness and pain in my chest diminished. It was not totally gone, but at least I could breathe without struggling. Satisfied that what was occurring in my chest was a passing situation, I went up to the kitchen. After refilling my cup, I proceeded up the stairs to my smoking lounge. There was some shortness of breath and discomfort breathing after climbing two flights of stairs, but nothing like the pain before. Stepping outside, I lit up again. After two puffs, it hit me. This time the pain in my chest was severe. It hit me like a bolt of lightning. I tried to breathe, but I couldn't. I gasped. It was all I could do to inhale. I had never felt anything like this before. I knew something was wrong, very wrong. I just didn't know what. Grinding out the cigarette, I went down to the kitchen. I called my wife, a registered nurse with many years of experience and I told her about the discomfort I was feeling in my chest. I tried to downplay the pain, but I suspect she picked up from my voice the intensity. By then it was all I could do to breathe and talk. I told her she needed to come home and take me to the emergency room.

She wouldn't hear of it. I was to hang up and immediately dial 911 for the Medic One ambulance. I told her that wasn't necessary, but she insisted that was what I needed to do, and I needed to do it right then. I said, "okay," and did what she instructed. By then I was really hurting. I told the 911 operator I was experiencing chest pains. She asked how much, and by then it was all I could do to talk. It was the worst pain I had ever felt. The 911 operator sensed from my voice the severity and told me to hold on. She was dispatching an emergency vehicle, and it would be to me momentarily.

By then I realized something was very wrong. I did not think it was a heart attack, as I had never had one of those before, but I was beginning to suspect that was the case. Seated at the base of the stairs, leading up to the kitchen and adjoining the great room above, I looked up when I heard our cat come racing down toward me. He took one sniff of me and promptly raced back up the stairs. At the top he turned and stared down at me. Even though cats have fewer facial muscles than humans, I could tell from his expression he was concerned, really concerned. Right then, I knew I was in trouble. If my cat could sense something was wrong, then something was seriously wrong.

Moments later, the fire department arrived. They did an immediate evaluation and promptly called for the Medic One unit. It took close to a half hour for the ambulance to arrive. There were multiple medical emergencies in the north end of Seattle that morning. The Emergency Medical Technician (EMT) gave me a shot of morphine. He said it would take a few minutes for it to dull the pain. It didn't. He gave me a second shot. That too, did little to squelch the burning in my chest. Following the third shot of morphine, the pain finally subsided. By then I was woozy. I was drifting in and out of awareness. I recall asking my neighbor, who had come over when he saw the fire truck, to lock up my house when they wheeled me out. I remembered that much and being loaded into the ambulance. The next thing I knew I was being wheeled into the emergency room.

The ER doctor checked me and asked me if I smoked. I said, "yes." He asked how much, and I answered, "two and a half packs a day." I downplayed the number since I smoked a full three packs daily. He had no other comment, and I was admitted. A couple of days later I awoke in a hospital bed. My wife, the RN, was standing beside me. She said I had gone through a couple of tough days. It turns out the cardiologist assigned to me had done an angiogram when I was first admitted. From that he concluded I had a plugged artery, and I needed a stent placed in the occlusion ASAP to open it up so the blood could once again flow freely. To do the procedure, insertion of the stent, he gave me a general anesthetic. I learned later, I reacted rather violently to that medication. When he made the incision in my groin to access a major artery and started sliding the probe up that artery toward my heart, I had become combative. To the extent he could not complete the procedure of placing a stent in the occluded portion of my heart artery. He was forced to retract the probe. He tried to wean me off the general anesthetic, which didn't work. I only became more violent. Unaware of how I had reacted to the anesthetic, my wife was shocked when she came to the hospital that evening to see me. When she saw I was strapped down to the bed, she exploded, as only a former hospital Director of Nursing can do. She ordered the restraints be removed immediately and she would care for her husband. She stayed with me until I was awake, lucid, and free of the anesthetic.

The cardiologist apologized for the anesthetic problem, but at the same time, reiterated that I needed the stent. My wife and I agreed, "fine, put in the stent be do it with a local anesthetic". The doctor retreated. He said he had never done the procedure under local anesthetic before. My wife and I said, "there was always a first time". The doctor pointed out that running a probe up an artery from the groin into the heart could be quite unsettling. He said there wouldn't be any feeling of the actual probe going up the artery, but the idea this tube was being pushed up me all the way into my heart could be very unnerving. "Stressful," I believe was the word he used. I said, "let me handle the stress," and he proceeded. I recall there was no pain or discomfort whatsoever. In fact, I didn't feel a thing. Throughout the whole process he kept asking me if I was feeling, "anything?" To which I answered, "no." He asked if I was, "okay?" and, I kept assuring him, "I was". When he got the probe to my heart he put in the stent, a short narrow tube inserted in an artery to keep it open. In as much as I was wide awake, he showed me the live x-ray image he was working by, of my heart. I saw the blockage and the probe and the stent. He described how, because of the artery blockage was rather extensive, it would be best if he put in a second stent, next to the one he just inserted, and I said, "go for it."

With two stents in place, I spent the next couple of days in the hospital recuperating. When it came time to be discharged, the cardiologist met with me to approve my release. He pointed out that I had been through a major event. Blockage of a heart artery is a significant event, considering my reaction to the original anesthetic compounded the problem. The good news was that I had made it through the initial heart attack and operation, and I was now on my way to recovery. With that, his discharge instructions were clear. He stated that with my weight at 232 pounds I was overweight. He said I needed to lose a good thirty pounds. I needed to get below 200. Added to that, he said I needed to STOP smoking. WHAT? I thought. I had smoked for over twenty-five years! I couldn't give up smoking. Cigarettes were a major part of my life. I smoked from the moment I got up to when I went to bed. I might consider cutting back a little, but quitting, no way. He also said I needed to start exercising. Ha, I thought, fat chance of me doing that. I hadn't exercised since I was in college and that had been years before. The last thing he said was that he needed to see me in his office in 30 days. He needed to check my cholesterol level and follow that with a stress test. *What?* I swallowed hard. "A stress test," I hesitantly asked. "Yes," he said. "A treadmill stress test," he replied. He was going to put me on his treadmill and check my heart rate, blood pressure and respiration.

That caught me off guard. A "stress test – on a treadmill no less?" I asked him what the treadmill test involved. He said it was standard procedure. He did a treadmill test on every patient following a heart attack. He said because it was the first test and only 30 days out of the hospital, he wasn't expecting much, but he would like to establish a baseline and see how far I could go on level one incline. He said that the first segment was five minutes. He smiled and said, "Don't worry about the five minutes. I only expect you to go as far as you feel comfortable and not be overtaxed." Again, he smiled. "Most patients only go a couple of minutes on level one, but that was enough for me to get a starting point," he stated. I asked, "What happened after that." He asked, "What do you mean?" I said, "After level one, what happens after that?" He frowned, "After level one I increase the angle of incline . . . another five degrees." I asked, "How long would that be for?" He said, "Five minutes," but I was not to be concerned about that as patients just 30 days out of the hospital, following a heart attack and the insertion of stents, never got to level two. "And if they did," I asked, "What then?" He shrugged and said there was level three where the treadmill incline would once again be increased. He smiled and said, "I could forget about level two and three as no one did them after only 30 days." He continued to smile in a calming way. I suspect to put me at ease. He continued. "In fact, few patients went the full five minutes of the level one incline." My cardiologist concluded by stating, following the first heart attack, average expectancy for another heart attack or the next event was six to eight years. When I heard that I immediately made it a goal to prove that average wrong. I was going to do everything in my power to extend that time between major cardiac events.

Following the pre-discharge meeting with the cardiologist, I was consumed with the hospital release process. I could not believe all the forms and paperwork I was presented with. Momentarily sweeping aside the cardiologist's instructions, and concern about the forth coming stress test, I was overjoyed, I was leaving the facility. And it was about time. I had seen enough of that sterile hospital environment and bland healthy meals, and I was ready to go home. I felt great. I felt I could leap the preverbal tall buildings with a single bound. Of course, the farthest I had walked since I had been admitted was from the bed to the adjoining bathroom and back, probably all ten feet each way, but that didn't matter. I felt fantastic. I could breathe. I had no chest pains. I was cured. I was ready to go home.

When the moment for me to leave arrived, the orderly came by my room with a wheelchair. I laughed and said I was healed and could walk to the exit. She stated it was hospital policy to wheel all discharged patients from their room to the exit. "Oh well, if you must," I said laughingly and was wheeled to street level. My wife had brought the car around and was parked across the drive lane from the exit. At the curb I told the orderly I was out of the hospital now and did not need the wheelchair anymore and could walk to the car on my own. Bounding to my feet, I felt great. I had been through a major medical procedure successfully and was ready to take on the world. Halfway across the drive lane, I faltered. My legs lost all strength. My knees buckled. Fortunately, the orderly was behind me. She grabbed me and assisted me into the chair when I started to fall. It turned out; I was not as recovered as I thought I was.

She helped me into the car, and I headed home. Minutes later, struggling from the car, I made it to the house. As soon as I walked through the front door, I wanted a cigarette. I had been without cigarettes for six days and could not wait to have a smoke. The heck with what the doctor had ordered, I was going to have a cigarette. To that end I asked my wife to go up to my smoking lounge and retrieve my smokes. She informed me there were no cigarettes in the house. "What!" I exclaimed. She went on to say, "there were no ashtrays and no lighters in the house either." Everything associated with cigarettes and smoking she had thrown away while I was in the hospital. If I wanted a pack, I would have to drive to the store and get it myself.

Exhaling loudly, I settled back on my heels. As much as I wanted a cigarette, I knew that was impossible. I didn't have the energy. It had been all I could do just getting from the car into the house, let alone drive anywhere and walk into a store. Shrugging my shoulders, I concluded if that is what my RN wife wanted, I would tough it out until I had the energy to get in the car and to the store on my own. I knew I should be able to do that in a couple of days.

Once at home I took a long look at myself. I could not believe what I saw . . . me, of all people had had a heart attack. How was that possible? I, like so many first-time heart-attack patients, was convinced heart attacks were something that happened to other people . . . heart attacks did not happen to them; but it had happened to me. Like it or not, the truth was, I had had a heart attack. I had coronary artery disease (CAD). That was the chilling reality, and I had no alternative but to accept that.

So, what was I going to do about heart disease? While recovering in the hospital I read all their literature about coronary artery disease. I learned the importance of weight control. I learned the importance of not smoking. While I did not hold out much hope for quitting cigarettes, I would at least give it a try. The exercise, I would work on that as soon as I got my strength back. The one thing I was going to do was do everything in my power to reduce the chances of another heart attack. The first one had been excruciatingly painful and frightening. I did not want to go through that horrible experience again, at least not any time soon.

But the fact was, I had had a heart attack. It turns out in the late 1990's I was one of roughly 210,000 people every month in the United States who have a heart attack. I was also one of a smaller number, roughly 140,000 who made it to the hospital in time and an even smaller number who survived that initial attack. I was lucky. Many do not survive the first heart attack. I had and to accomplish that several very skilled people got me through that first hospitalization phase, and to them I will be eternally grateful. But my road to recovery didn't end there, in fact that was only the beginning.

In the process of reading about heart disease, heart attacks, as well as the causes and the preventive steps I should have taken to have avoided that initial attack, I also learned if I already had that initial attack, how to reduce the probability of having a second attack. To me that was especially important. Experiencing that chest pain and the follow-on initial stay in the hospital was enough. I had my wakeup call, and it was now time to act.

For those of you who have had a heart attack and are reading this, the good news is you're still alive. As in my case, several people worked hard to pull me through and together we won. I faced a tough situation and am now over the worst. I was on the road to recovery, and it was time to move ahead.

So, what do I need to do now? Having had a heart attack and having been diagnosed with heart disease, CAD, a moment of reflection was a good place to start. I told myself it was time to take a step back and take a long look at what I had done and what I should not have done. While in the hospital I read the literature handed out about heart disease and heart attacks. In short order, I got down on myself for having a heart attack in the first place. How could I have been so stupid to allow myself to have a heart attack? I don't know how I did, but I did. That much was a given. As hard as that was to admit, nothing was going to reverse reality. Therefore, I had no other choice but to move ahead.

Now was the time to take that first step on the road back. I could not ignore the past. I had to learn from it to keep from experiencing another attack. I had to look honestly at what I had done to cause the CAD and heart attack in the first place and how to move forward from there. Even though I was only days out of the hospital, it was time to start. This was not something I could put off and start fresh on the first of the next month or some convenient time after that. No sir! The time to begin moving ahead and working on reducing the chance of a follow-on event, or second heart attack was right then. Moving ahead meant progressing toward a long, richer, fulfilling life; the kind that just a few days before, when I was riding in that ambulance to the hospital, was a fleeting dream.

Buoyed by the fact a healthy life didn't have to be a faraway dream; I told myself I could prevail; I could overcome this Coronary Heart Disease. Right then I made up my mind I would do whatever was necessary to accomplish that better life. As I told myself, "I've had my wake-up call. Don't let that initial pain and mental anguish go to waste. Now is the time to move ahead."

The first thing I knew I had to do was sit down alone and think about what caused my heart attack, or heart disease in the first place and get that phase over with. That I needed to do, and I needed to do that alone. Right then I didn't need a room full of well-meaning relatives and friends hammering on me about everything they were so sure I had done wrong and what they were positive I needed to do to correct my errant ways.

So, I took a few minutes to look at what I had been doing that brought on the heart disease and consequential heart attack. Unfortunately, it was chilling. However, I had to address what I had been doing wrong before I could correct my past behavior and start moving forward.

What I saw was a guy in his late fifties who had been forty-plus pounds overweight for decades. I saw a guy who smoked sixty-plus cigarettes a day, who ate fat-laden junk foods, and considered a walk to his car exercise. That was a recipe for disaster. I had dug myself a big hole to crawl out of, but that was minor compared to the first big challenge I faced, namely I had to admit to myself I had heart disease. That's right. Even with the chest pain still vivid in my mind and the hospital experience imprinted on my brain, openly accepting the fact I had a heart attack was difficult to do, and it continued to be so for several months after that. Looking back, I realized that was not a point or issue to dwell upon. A heart attack had occurred. There was no erasing history. I now had to focus on the future and how to minimize the chances of having another, and possibly a fatal heart attack. That was something in my control.

The *WHEN* to start on this road to recovery was, right THEN! The *HOW* was the more difficult part. To fully recover, I would have to start exercising gradually, and I would have to do right away. I could not put it off, for just the right day, when the weather was perfect or the temperatures were the most comfortable. I had to do it right **then**!

What immediately came to mind was what all my friends and relatives kept saying to me. In a common voice, they insisted I should take it easy. I should not overexert myself. After all I had heart disease and had a heart attack and didn't want to have another. To a degree, my doctor agreed. He phrased it differently though, saying I should start out gradually. I should do for myself as my strength and endurance would allow. My doctor said that I should not let everyone do everything for me. He stressed I should not become a heart attack invalid. He said I could let the 'well meaning' friends and relatives initially help with the strenuous tasks, but I should gradually wean them off from doing that as my strength started to recover and build. And he said, my strength would recover, it would just take time.

When I first got home from the hospital, it took a few days for me to recover enough climb the one flight of stairs from the bedroom level to the kitchen. I would take it one step at a time, resting between steps, but I was determined to get up there on my own. I wasn't going to make my wife bring my meals down from the floor above. So, I took a step and stopped, then another step and stopped, until I eventually made it to the top. Looking back, that was quite an accomplishment. I was making progress progress—enough progress to start looking ahead. What immediately came to mind was that dreaded stress test the cardiologist wanted me to take in his office in 4 weeks.

Right then, I knew I had my work cut out for me. Deep down, I wanted to prove to my doctor —and everyone else—that I hadn't suffered as severe a heart attack as they believed, or at least not the catastrophic event they made it out to be. Although I couldn't undo the past, I now had an extra motivation correct some of my errant ways During my hospital discharge visit, I asked my doctor if it would be okay to exercise once I got home. His response was specific and to the point, "NO! Working out with weights or anything strenuous was out of the question.

I asked him, "What about walking?" "Walking," he said was "okay." He advised me to wait a few days for my endurance and energy to recover some and then to start with short walks of a block or so at first but to do it, walk. He also insisted, "NO CIGARETTES!" unless I wanted to be right back in the hospital with another heart attack. And the next one could be fatal. Not good. The doctor pointed out that it would take about five years for my lungs to clear themselves of the effects of smoking, but they would if I never had another cigarette. The last thing he stated was about my weight. While in the hospital, I had dropped eight pounds in six days. That wasn't a good endorsement for hospital food. All the same, losing eight pounds was a start. It was the first step in peeling off the thirty-plus pounds to get below 200.

It was clear that exercise—or more specifically, walking—was only part of the solution; in fact, it was only one-fourth of the equation. Another big issue was my smoking habit. A three-pack-a-day addiction was going to be tough to break, but I had to quit if I hoped to tackle my heart disease. My doctor admant: I couldn't just cut my smoking in half to a pack and a half a day —I had to stop completely. Even a couple of cigarettes a day would still harm my lungs and make my heart work harder. Quitting entirely was the only option. To that end, my wife helped. While I was in the hospital she had gone around the house and got rid of all my smoking paraphernalia. She figured, "Out of sight, out of mind." And it worked. At first, I was too tired to consider driving to the store to buy a pack. Over the two days I'd been home from the hospital without cigarettes, I noticed something unexpected: I wasn't grouchy. The desire for a cigarette had diminished from an outright insatiable need to a feeling resembling a bad food craving. I was not over smoking but to my amazement with each passing day, the desire became less intense. Initially, when I got an almost irresistible urge to smoke, I forced myself to recall the excruciating chest pain I experienced during the heart attack. And let me tell you, the pain was intense. To help take my mind off the urge for a cigarette, I would step outside and go for even a short walk. All be it brief, out to the street and back, or a hundred or so feet up the hill, but a walk all the same. I discovered that breathing deeply during that short stroll was refreshing. Everything had begun to smell great, the trees, the flowers, even the air itself. I was enjoying fragrances I hadn't sensed for over 35 years. I couldn't believe it. I was quitting the smoking habit.

Walking was the next of the doctor's requirements I chose to tackle. After recuperating in the house for a couple of days I decided I better start walking more than a couple hundred feet. I live in a cove, and my house sits on the side of a hill that is quite steep. It seemed like every direction from my house was up. The closest intersection was about a hundred-foot climb up a rather steep incline. I remembered looking up the hill and thinking, "There's no time like the present to get started – so let's do it." Taking one step at a time, I trudged up those hundred feet to the first cross street. It took me ten minutes and I was winded up when I got to the intersection, but I was there. Looking back, while debating what to do next, I realized that while I was breathing deeply, I wasn't out of breath.

I was possibly less winded than I would have been if I had taken the same walk before my heart attack. While on cigarettes I could not have made that one-hundred-foot hill climb. Being off cigarettes for little over a week had already had an effect, a positive effect.

Feeling good, I looked back. To my amazement, I had made it up a steep grade. Ahead of me, the street was more gradual, so I thought, "Why not? Go for it." I figured I would take it easy and if I got tired, the way back to my house would be all downhill. To my delight, I made it to the far end of the development, next to where I lived. It had been a long trudge, but I had made it. Turning around, I headed back to my house. Days later I measured how far that distance was I had walked that first day. It was six-tenths of a mile to the end of the development. I had done the 1.2 miles round trip, in a bit over an hour. The next morning, I did the same walk, this time though I did the 1.2-mile walk in an hour. Unbelievably, one week out of the hospital, I had just walked further than I had walked in the previous 35 years. Each day, the walk became easier. By the time the first doctor's appointment rolled around for that initial stress test, I was doing the 1.2 miles in just under a half hour.

The third thing I had to tackle was the cholesterol test. This time my wife, the RN stepped forward. Not knowing exactly what I wanted to eat when I came home from the hospital, nor how much time she might have to cook, she picked out some '*heart healthy,*' frozen meals from the store to see if one of them might pique my interest. Initially, I told her, "Just heat it. It couldn't taste worse than hospital food. To my amazement, those frozen, '*heart healthy*' meals were quite tasty. Not only were they appetizing, but they were also very filling. While in the hospital I learned the importance of a correct diet. Not only about what to eat as well as when to eat. A balanced diet starts with eating three meals a day. That did not mean a large cup of coffee or cappuccino for breakfast, donuts and more coffee for lunch, and a huge, fat-laden, high-calorie oversized meal for dinner. In my case, that was very true. For decades I never ate breakfast I didn't have the time. For lunch, I would grab whatever was convenient from a fast-food drive-through window and hit it big for dinner.

I thought, oh well, I would give the three meal a day scenario a try. I figured all I had to lose was weight. I would start by focusing on what I ate. I would also control my intake of fat and sugar. The literature stressed, "control your fat and sugar intake and you can take charge of your weight." An interesting thought, that I hoped was right. Following the advice in the literature, I began eating breakfast, a bowl of dry cereal with fat free milk. Turns out cold cereal was not just for kids, but adults could enjoy it as well. Next was lunch, which consisted of a sandwich with lean meat on whole-wheat bread, low-fat baked potato chips, a low-fat cookie or two, and water to drink. Dinner was one of those 'heart-healthy, low-fat meals, my wife had picked out and a Jello or similar low-fat dessert.

A couple of days later, I checked my weight and to my amazement, I weighed 10 pounds less than I did the morning before my heart attack. I couldn't believe it. During the previous 20+ years, I had tried practically every way to lose weight and had never lost more than 5 pounds. The worst part was, I had never kept the weight off. Now, eating three meals a day, and walking every morning, I had lost an extra four pounds. What progress? What reinforcement? My new eating habits, diet, and exercise were working.

Now the next hurdle - that dreaded stress test on the treadmill. From the moment I had enough energy to start walking, I did. At first at a slow pace. I started doing the 1.2-mile round trip in a leisure one hour plus. Day by day I worked on bringing that time down. By the third week, I was down to just under 25 minutes. I was bound and determined to do well on the treadmill. By the end of the fourth week, I had stretched the distance to a 1.5-mile round trip.

Thirty days following discharge from the hospital was the date for my first cardiologist visit. A week before I was to go in for the treadmill test, I had stopped by the lab and had blood drawn for a cholesterol check. Upon entering the doctor's office, in week four he began by going over the laboratory results. He was pleased to say that my cholesterol readings were all within normal ranges. There was nothing there to raise any red flags.

Next, it was time to do the treadmill. Level one was at the lowest incline, but it was an incline and not a level. I started walking at the steady pace of the moving surface. It was brisk, but not tiring. In fact, by the end of the first five minutes, I had no trouble keeping up. At the end of the first five minutes, the cardiologist asked if felt I could go further. He pointed out that the incline of the walking surface would be increased an additional 5 degrees, Proud that I had made it through the first level without breathing hard, I agreed to continue. The doctor increased the angle of the incline. And yes, it took more energy, and I was breathing deeper, but I was not out of breath. Throughout the second level of incline, the doctor kept asking if I was getting short of breath and wanted to stop. I said, "No", and for him to raise the walking surface to the next level of incline. The doctor said he would if I wanted to give it a try and I said, "Yes." Two and a half minutes into level three, the doctor said he had seen enough, and the treadmill test was concluded. He asked me how I did it, and how did I go to the third level. I told him I was determined to make it to level three and beyond if I needed to. I didn't tell him that deep down I was determined to prove to myself that the heart attack I experienced had not been severe and that it had been mild, which it wasn't. An artery had been completely blocked and that was a fact. I know it was impossible to prove my heart attack had not been severe, because the pain had been very strong and gripping, but still, in my own mind, I felt if I could get to level three that would somehow signal to me that I hadn't had a major heart attack event.

The doctor acknowledged he could not recall any 30-day post-heart attack person making it into level three of the treadmill. He stated that very few of his patients made it much past two minutes or to the halfway point of level one, let alone into level two. He asked me what I had done to prepare for the test, and I told him I had started walking. I was doing 1.2 miles every morning and had just increased that to 2 full miles the day before. He was pleased with my progress and said to me not to stop.

That I did and within six months I was up to 6 miles a day. It took me a couple of months, but I got up to where I could do the 6 miles in a consistent hour and a half. I was walking at a steady four-mile-per-hour pace, uphill, downhill, rain or shine. I continued doing that for the next sixteen-plus years. That accomplishment forestalled my next heart attack event and lessened the severity of it in the process.

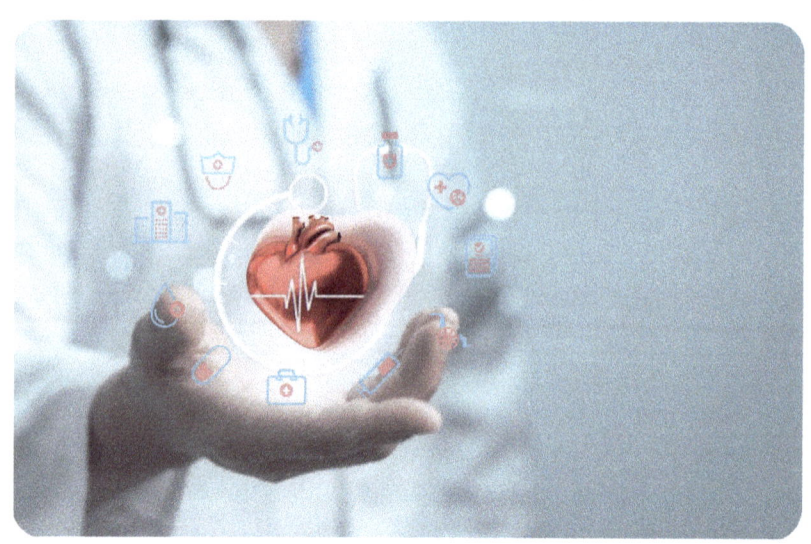

Chapter 2

L ying in the hospital, following that first heart attack, I was scared. What was my fate? I didn't know what to expect. Where do I go from here? I didn't want to die. I had a wife and children. I had much to live for. I had to figure out a way to move ahead. I had to whip this thing called heart disease.

I quickly realized the person most interested in my battle with heart disease and with my recovery from the heart attack was me. That's right. The ultimate responsibility fell on my shoulders. While my doctor and wife and family members were quite concerned about getting me well, responsibility for my long-term recovery and health was with me. To do so didn't mean I would have to become as schooled and knowledgeable as my doctor, but the more I knew about my illness, coronary artery disease, and the correct path to recovery, the more likely I was to follow the specifics laid out by my doctors and care providers to live a long productive life. After all my initial heart attack was a 'wake-up call' and not a 'death sentence'. To move ahead I realized the more I knew and the more I learned, the better off I would be. Also, the more I learned about heart disease, the more relieved I became and the less I feared the disease and the possible future attack. So I set about putting together a list of additional questions I needed to answer to better understand my illness and the probability of a long healthy life. Below are the more significant questions I initially came up with and what I learned.

#1. How severe was my heart disease? That was good to know. Was it mild and a wake-up call as I was hoping, and something I needed to follow or was my heart attack a forewarning of a possible severe event that was ahead and was a signal that my time was measured?

I went so far as to have my cardiologist show me a diagram of the heart where exactly the blood flow restriction occur and how large was the affected area. Was the heart attack because of that blockage and damage; mild, medium, or severe? My cardiologist outlined the area of my heart that had been affected. At the time I could not believe how such a small, damaged area could have produced so much pain. He pointed out that even a confined area like that can produce an extreme amount of pain. He also stated that while every heart attack was a major event because the area of my heart that was affected was localized, with proper medical attention, diet, and exercise, a long healthy life was possible.

2. One of my next questions concerned blood pressure. That the doctor would check with every appointment. That opened the door for many more questions. If it were high, what would it be? What can I do to bring it into the accepted range? If it were low, what was the significance of that? Can that be a life-threatening situation? Is there anything I can do about 'low blood' pressure?

My cardiologist gave me a couple of prescriptions. I asked what they were for and how long I would need to take them. The later question he answered simply, "forever". When I asked what they were for, he gave me a brief canned answer, "Blood pressure," and he said little else. I asked if they should be taken with food or on an empty stomach and he said that didn't make any difference and if there were the label on the bottle coming from the pharmacy would so state. I asked if there were side effects, and he said he had been prescribing these for years and none of his patients had complained of any problems or complications.

I asked if it was okay to take the prescribed medication with the other medications that had been prescribed by my family doctor. He reviewed the list of medications and over-the-counter supplements I was taking and said they wouldn't create a problem with what he prescribed.

I asked him how often I should have my cholesterol checked, and he said yearly, prior to my annual visit to see him. I asked about alcohol, and he said in moderation. He said a glass or so of wine and one cocktail was allowed.

Aside from the above, I asked if there were any other restrictions and he said I could keep doing what I had been doing to lose weight; namely watching my diet, my weight and exercising daily.

Following that visit I picked up everything I could find to read about heart attacks, heart disease, and coronary artery disease. The more I read the more questions I had. Everything was becoming a blur. I couldn't call my cardiologist every time I didn't understand some word or statement. He was way too busy to be bothered with an endless stream of inquiries. Whereupon it became obvious finding the answers to my questions fell on my shoulders. I decided every time I didn't know something, I would research that until I found out what it meant in straight-forward words, and not in erudite terms that only educated physicians and medical personnel could understand. I wanted to know what the questions I had meant in common, everyday language. With time on my hands, during the recovery phase, I pursued my quest for information.

To begin with, what exactly is your heart? We all know the heart is an organ that pumps blood around the body. Fine. But what is it really? A human heart is a phenomenal muscular organ about the size of a fist. It has two sides, a left side and a right side. Each side has two chambers: an upper chamber and a lower chamber. The four chambers are the upper right chamber or right atrium. The lower right chamber or ventricle. The upper left chamber or left atrium and the lower left chamber or left ventricle. There are four valves controlling the flow of blood in and out of the heart and between the four chambers. The valves are the 'Tricuspid Valve', the 'Pulmonary Valve', the 'Mitral Valve', and the 'Aortic Valve'. Blood comes into the heart from the body via the vena cava into the upper right chamber (atrium). The oxygen depleted blood then passes into the right ventricle (lower right chamber) where it is pumped to the lungs. Passing through the lungs the blood picks up oxygen. The oxygen rich blood coming back from the lungs enters the upper left chamber (left atrium). The oxygenated blood then passes into the left ventricle where it is pumped out into the body. This process repeats itself with no conscious input on the part of the human roughly 72 times a minute which equates to 4,320 times per hour, and 103,680 times per day, 725,760 beats per week, and so on. The heart muscle, like the rest of the body, requires an uninterrupted supply of oxygen rich blood to perform its pumping action and that blood is provided by the arteries surrounding the heart, the coronary arteries. If one or more of the coronary arteries becomes occluded, or plugged, and stops the flow of oxygen to the heart muscle, that is what causes the pain, when a portion of the heart muscle tissue is starved of oxygen. That is a heart attack. In my case the pain was severe.

Next came the terms, and words that are so frequently associated with heart disease and stroke. One of the most frequently used words is cholesterol. We hear that word used every day, but what does it mean? What is cholesterol? What is it composed of? Where does it come from? How does it affect the body? Is all cholesterol bad for us? How can we live with cholesterol? Can we control or reduce the effects of cholesterol and if so, how? This I will go into in-depth and answer.

I was overweight, but by how much? What should I weigh? What is the optimum body weight for a person of my height, frame size, and age? How is it determined? What is this term that has become the buzzword, BMI – Body Mass Index? What does it mean?

Following a heart attack, I was supposed to exercise. What exercises are approved and what are not? What exercises will put an unacceptable strain on my heart and what exercises won't? Can I work out with weights? Can I jog? Can I ride a bike? Can I run, and if so, how much? These were all questions I needed answers to. Of the approved exercises, how many calories are burned with each type of activity? What are Activity Factors? What exactly is coronary artery disease (CAD). Is there a cure for CAD?

What are the accepted ranges for blood pressure? What blood pressure is considered too high and what is considered too low? What exactly is blood pressure? What are accepted Pulse rates? What is considered too high or rapid a pulse and what is considered too low. What is considered approved pulse rates with the different forms of exercise?

Foods? What foods are considered heart-healthy and which ones are not? What types of foods should I avoid?

Alcohol, can I have a drink? If so, how much? How often? Is wine acceptable?

Cigarettes. Are any allowed? If so, how many per day is allowed or do I have to quit altogether? Are e-cigarettes safe? Are they allowed?

When can I start exercising? What is Angina? Is angina a death sentence? How can I identify Angina if it occurs? How can I tell Angina from a heart attack? If Angina does occur, what should I do?

And the list goes on and on. These were all the things I needed answers to. The more I got into my studies, the more I realized I needed to know a lot to control, or at least live with coronary artery disease (CAD). In the end, living with CAD became my goal.

Below is some of what I learned following my initial heart attack. Mind you, we can never cure or overcome CAD or heart disease. But we can learn how to not fear heart disease and live with CAD (coronary artery disease) and make the most out of the days ahead and extend our lives as much as possible.

Cholesterol: one of the many governments reports I read, indicated that roughly 42 million Americans had high cholesterol and that 63 million more Americans had borderline high cholesterol. In 2016 the US Department of Agriculture recommended that Americans eat as little dietary cholesterol as possible. Left alone, the body will produce the cholesterol it needs. The USDA advocated Americans reduce the cholesterol in their bodies through changes in diet as well as lifestyle modifications.

So, what is this thing called cholesterol? It turns out cholesterol is a waxy substance the body needs to build and replace cells. Really? Which means cholesterol is naturally occurring in human bodies. At the correct levels of cholesterol, everything is in balance and the body works just fine. Too much cholesterol though, can be a problem. Cholesterol in the body comes from two sources, the liver which produces roughly 80% of all the cholesterol the body needs, and the body's intestines, adrenal glands, and reproductive organs which produce the rest. In addition to those natural sources, cholesterol also comes from animal foods, specifically meats, poultry, and full-fat-laden dairy products. These foods are high in saturated fats and trans fats. Ingestion of these fats causes the body (specifically the liver) to make more cholesterol than it otherwise needs, which in turn can cause the body to go from a normal balanced cholesterol level to an unhealthy, unbalanced, elevated level. In addition to meat, poultry, and fatty dairy products, tropical oils such as palm oils, coconut oil and palm kernel oils (commonly found in baked goods) can also signal the liver to make more cholesterol than the body needs for normal cell production and replacement.

There are two types of cholesterol. The two types are commonly referred to 'LDL' and 'HDL'. What exactly are they and what do the letters mean? LDL (low density lipoprotein) is the major blood cholesterol carrier, which is frequently referred to as 'the bad cholesterol' when found in excess. In excess concentrations LDL can and will deposit its excess waxy particles on the walls of arteries, thereby causing the inside of the artery to narrow and become less flexible in a process called atherosclerosis. When that buildup blocks or forms a clot in an artery that is when a heart attack or stroke can, and frequently occurs. In my case, that buildup completely blocked one of the arteries around my heart which resulted in excruciating discomfort and pain.

The other main type of cholesterol is HDL (high density lipoprotein), which is frequently referred to as 'good cholesterol'. This good cholesterol works to pick up LDL and transport the excess LDL back to the liver for reprocessing and excretion; thereby reducing the LDL level.

The American Heart Association (AHA) and other health-minded Cholesterol education groups have recommended that the results of a blood cholesterol test, following a total 12 hour fasting period prior to the test, should be as follows: normal blood cholesterol levels, need to be below 200 mg/dl. Borderline-high-risk cholesterol levels are listed as between 200 mg/dl to 239 mg/dl. Collectively, they have stated cholesterol levels above 240 mg/dl be classified as high risk and an increased cardiovascular disease mortality rate. Not good. Even though AHA and other groups state that good LDL levels be below 200 mg/dl, for increased health, they really say LDL should be at or below 130 mg/dl with a ratio of LDL to HDL be 5:1 or less to be healthier.

The frequency of having 12-hour fasting cholesterol tests varies with each physician. There are mitigating circumstances that only the physician is aware of to determine when a test is required. I go into more detail about Cholesterol in Chapter 7.

Another question that came to mind following my original heart attack was **Blood Pressure**. When I went home my cardiologist told me to get a blood pressure cuff, one of those you put around your wrist to measure blood pressure. He also wanted me to keep a daily record of my blood pressure and pulse rate, for the next few months and to bring that record with me during my future visits. That immediately brought up some questions. What exactly is 'blood pressure?' It is a term we all use but what is it? Blood pressure, it turns out, is the pressure the circulating blood exerts on the artery walls while flowing through your body. Following my first heart attack, when I was doing my initial research to find answers to my questions there was no on-line resource Wikipedia, as Jimmy Wales and Larry Sanger did not create that online source until January 15, 2001. What I learned was that blood pressure readings are composed of two values. A high pressure or '**systolic**', pressure when the blood is forced (pumped) out of the heart, and the lower pressure or '**diastolic**' pressure, when the blood returns to the heart. These pressure values are measured in millimeters of mercury (mmHg) above the normal atmospheric pressure surrounding the body. Over the years normal blood pressure for a middle-aged adult is considered 120 mmHg, systolic pressure, and 80 mmHg, diastolic pressure. There are many extraneous factors that cause fluctuations in those 'high' (systolic) and 'low' (diastolic) pressure readings such as stress, both physical and emotional; health, mainly if the person suffers from some form of trauma such as major sickness or injury; age is also a factor, as is, is the person on drugs, both legal and otherwise. Smoking is also a major factor as smoking constricts the blood vessels thereby causing the heart to pump harder to move the blood through the body. Smoking also coats the lungs with secretions reducing the surface area in the lungs for oxygen to be transferred to the blood, thereby causing the heart to pump more blood through the lungs to get oxygenated.

The commonly accepted blood pressure reading for a person over 20 years old are:

	Systolic	Diastolic
Normal	90 mmHg – 119 mmHg	60 mmHg – 79 mmHg
Pre-hypertensive	120 mmHg – 129 mmHg	60 mmHg – 79 mmHg
Hypertensive	140 mmHg – 159 mmHg	90 mmHg – 99 mmHg
Serious Hypertensive	>greater than 160 mmHg	> greater than 100 mmHg

If pressure readings are above 'serious hypertensive', that is a reason to seek medical attention. The incidence of a heart attack and stroke increases with those elevated pressures. Pressure readings below the 'normal' readings are also caused to consult a physician.

Two words that come up when monitoring blood pressure are '**Hypotension**' or low blood pressure. When systolic blood pressure is less than 90 mmHg, and or diastolic pressure is less than 60 mmHg that is considered low and cause to contact a cardiologist, as pressures much below that can result in dizziness, fainting spells and an indication of possible heart disorders.

Likewise, '**Hypertension**' or high systolic pressure in the range of 120 mmHg – 139 mmHg and diastolic pressure in the range of 70 mmHg – 89 mmHg is cause for concern indicating attention needs to be paid to lifestyle, cholesterol, and weight as well as smoking. Systolic pressure from 140 mmHg – 179 mmHg and diastolic pressure in the range of 90 mmHg – 109 mmHg is cause for monitoring and treatment by a physician. Systolic pressure at or above 180 mmHg and diastolic at or above 120 mmHg is approaching crisis level and requires immediate medical attention.

Another term was '**Angina**'. What exactly is angina? Angina is discomfort in the center of the chest lasting many minutes and characterized by a feeling of heaviness or pressure on the chest that comes about following exertion, strenuous exercising such as running, or even following a full meal or exposure to sudden cold temperatures. If the discomfort is relieved by resting and stopping what you were doing and lying down and relaxing for a few minutes that indicates it was probably angina, a temporary reduction of blood flow to the heart. If the discomfort reoccurs when the physical activity is continued, that is also an indication of angina. If following stopping the activity and resting the pain persists and does not subside that is caused to consider medical assistance. If the discomfort is accompanied by chest pain, then it is best to seek immediate medical attention as this could mean you are experiencing a heart attack (a myocardial infarction).

Factors increasing the occurrence of angina include smoking cigarettes, high blood pressure, elevated cholesterol, and a sedentary lifestyle preceding strenuous physical activity. Age is another contributing factor. With age comes an increase in the probability of experiencing angina as the blood vessels surrounding the heart are less flexible and do not compensate as easily following exertion.

If the occurrence of angina persists and repeats every few weeks that is an indication there possibly is a greater heart issue that needs to be addressed and seeing a cardiologist is strongly recommended.

I will go into more detail about Angina in Chapter 9.

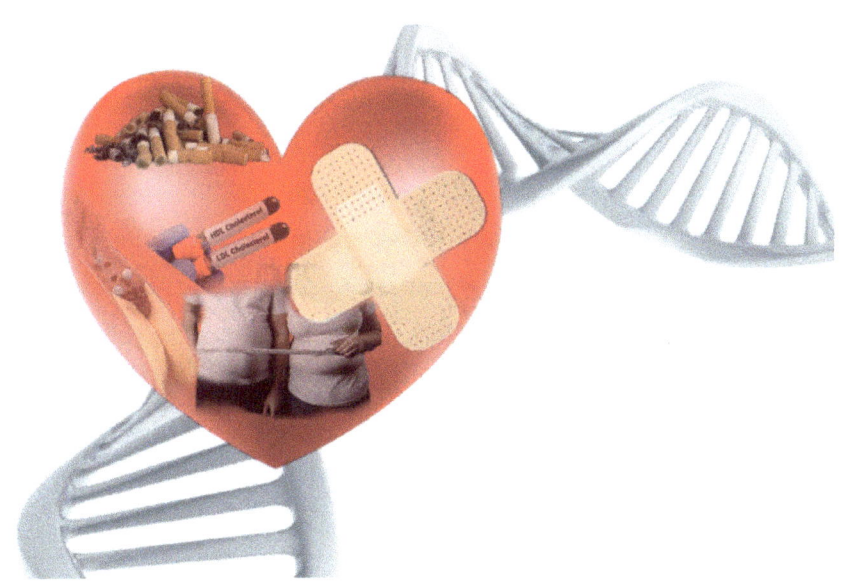

Chapter 3

Factors that increased a risk of a heart attack or stroke.

Back in the late 1990's when I had my initial heart attack, I discovered I belonged to a big club, in fact, a very big club that was growing by the day. In the United States, at that time, it was growing at the rate of 208,333 on average per month, or the frightening rate of about two and a half million new heart attack patients per year. But that was nothing compared to the alarming statistic, upwards of 20% of the population suffered from some form of heart disease, not just in the United States but worldwide. A diagnosis of heart disease can be viewed in a couple of ways. It can be viewed as a '*wakeup call*' to improve your health and lifestyle, or a '*death sentence*'. I preferred the former, *'wakeup call'*. I had survived the initial heart attack, now it was time to get smart.

A famous sage once said, a key to a long life was to have experienced a serious illness so you are forced to live within the restrictions that come about from that illness. How true that was. Hundreds of thousands of people who have had a heart attack, or the predisposing condition for a heart attack and are still with us are living proof of that. Live within the restrictions, and constraints associated with a diagnosis of coronary artery disease and life will go on and frequently better. In essence, I had faced our maker and now know what to do.

To begin with, I reviewed the factors that contributed to my developing heart disease. This was what I called my reality check. That was hard to do. Sometimes facing reality is difficult, but it had to be done before I could move ahead. Taking that hard cold look at the facts was chilling, but it had to be done. No one wants to admit what they did was wrong, especially wrong enough to create a life-threatening situation. I know I didn't, but as I discovered, it was important to honestly admit how I had brought this illness upon myself. Once I recognized the factors that contributed to my heart attack, the mending process began.

Factor number one, is **AGE**. Obviously, that was something over which I had no control, but age was a contributing factor. The age-related factors are; if you are a male over 45, you are entering that age range when the risks from heart disease and heart attacks are more likely to occur. In other words, over 45 we need to become aware of the other factors, we can control that contribute to heart disease and see what we can do to reduce their significance. For women, the age warning factor comes into play when they pass 55, have completed menopause or have had their ovaries removed and are not on estrogen replacement therapy.

The above **Age Factors** are not contributing conditions to spawn heart disease by itself, but when combined with other the factors listed below, should give cause to note, or at least become more aware of the increase in the risk of developing heart disease. The main takeaway point, the risk of having a heart attack goes up with age. This is known as the caution area. In my case, I was 59 at the time, well in that danger zone.

Family History. For men, if your father or brother had a heart attack before the age of 55, that is a factor to be considered. For women, if your mother or sister had a heart attack before 65, then take note. For me, my brother had a heart attack in his early fifties and my mother suffered from high blood pressure and had a stroke by age 57. All negative signs.

Obesity. An affliction effects between a third to half of the population; depending on what study I read. If a person is 20 or more pounds overweight, combined with one or more contributing factors, that too could increase the probability of a heart attack. In my case, I was 45 pounds overweight, and though I had tried to lose weight, I had never lost and kept off even a couple of pounds.

Physical Activity. More correctly stated, physical inactivity. Physical inactivity is a major contributing factor toward increasing the risk of having a heart attack. The heart is a muscular organ and is only as strong as it must work. If a person lives a very sedate or inactive life, the heart is never exercised. When a demand is placed on the heart that the heart is not accustomed to, the heart can fail. That failure is called a heart attack. Again, in my case, I had to come to grips with the fact I considered walking up a flight of stairs 50 + times a day to get to my cigarette exercise. Beyond that, I did little exercise other than walking to and from my car.

Cholesterol: An additional factor. If *Total* cholesterol is 240 mg/dl or higher, that is a major factor in increasing the risk of a heart attack. Chances are for those who eat a junk food diet high in fats, their cholesterol is elevated, possibly through the roof. Again, my case. However total cholesterol is made up of several components. As described earlier, one of the components is HDL, the good cholesterol. If the HDL, or good cholesterol, is less than 35 mg/dl, that is bad. HDL needs to be above 35 mg/dl. Below that can be a contributing factor for an increased risk of heart disease and a heart attack.

Smoking. A major factor. Studies indicate that even smoking only a few cigarettes a day is bad. Smoking 2 to 3 packs a day is inviting disaster. A fact I discovered after my heart attack; more smokers die of heart disease, namely heart attacks, than all forms of lung disease; even lung cancer. Smoking even the lowest tar and nicotine cigarette is no less good for you than the highest tar and nicotine cigarette. Tar and nicotine are just that, tar and nicotine, period.

The three contributing factors to smoking, are:

1. The nicotine component of smoking narrows the blood vessels causing the heart to work harder to push the blood through the body's narrowed passageways, two puffs of a cigarette, even the mildest cigarette, will cause the blood vessels to restrict, (narrow) for up to twenty minutes. If two puffs can do that it is not hard to see what the effect of ten, twenty or more cigarettes will be.

2. Smoking adds carbon monoxide to the lungs which has a double barrel effect. One, it causes secretions to form. Those secretions coat the inside of the lungs, reducing the surface area available to transfer oxygen to the blood. Second, the less oxygen transferred to the blood, the more the heart must work to pump the oxygen poor blood around the system to satisfy the body's need for oxygen.

3. **Carbon Monoxide**. With smoking comes an increase in the carbon monoxide levels in the lungs. The carbon monoxide displaces oxygen, resulting in less oxygen in the lungs for the blood to capture. With less oxygen in the lungs for the red cells in the blood to pick up, the heart again, must work harder. The heart is forced to pump more blood through the lungs to pick up what little oxygen is there to feed the cells in the body. A never-ending problem.

The word to smokers is **STOP**. As every smoker will attest to, that is easier said than done. Those who have tried to quit smoking have frequently tried everything and cannot shake the habit. There are any number of packaged products, pills, and capsules on the market that supposedly will help the smoker break their dependency. Wrong. Pills substitute one habit for another. The easiest way to quit the smoking habit is to just stop. I know that sounds impossible, but it is true. In my case, the 6 days I was in the hospital, I did not have a cigarette. When I got home, my wife had thrown away all the cigarettes, the ashtrays, lighters, and matches. I couldn't smoke if I wanted to. At the same time, I did not have the strength to go to the store myself, so I did the next best thing, I rested. I did not have the energy to get in my car and drive to the store. So, I had no choice but to not smoke. When I started to get my energy back, I had been off cigarettes for close to 2 weeks. If I could do it for 2 weeks, I should be able to keep off cigarettes another day or two longer. Little by little, the days started to add up and became a week. One week off cigarettes grew into two and then three and then a month and so on. Whenever I would get the insatiable urge to have a cigarette, I would go for a walk until the urge disappeared. As it turned out with the passage of time the urge to smoke became less. I discovered I was enjoying the smells of nature that I had been missing for all those years. If that wasn't enough to deter me from buying a pack and lighting up, I would think about the excruciating chest pain I had experienced with that heart attack, which was still vividly imprinted in my memory, and how I never wanted to experience that again, and suddenly the urge to light up went away.

Blood Pressure: Another factor that increases the probability of developing heart disease and the subsequent heart attack is high blood pressure. This runs a close second to smoking contributing factors for heart attacks. If at rest blood pressure is above 140/90 mm Hg, that is considered elevated or high and is a major heart disease contributing factor. High blood pressure is and can be controlled by several well-tested pharmaceutical products that are safe and reduce blood pressure. Blood pressure is one of the first things that is checked when you visit a doctor's office or hospital. It is that important, and one of the easier physical conditions to manage.

For me, most of the factors listed above were present prior to my original heart attack. So, to move ahead I had to take control of my life. To begin with I could place 'age' and 'family history' aside. Those were the factors over which I had no control. That left me with the factors over which I had influence and control and manage them I must do.

Controlling my weight was a good place to start, which brought up the question, how much should I weigh. Really, how should I or how could I determine, with some degree of accuracy, how much should I weigh? As it turned out, that is a question that frequently invokes as many different answers as people offer them. To help answer the question about how to calculate a person's ideal weight based on age and frame size I have gone into depth to describe the more generally accepted methods in the next chapter, chapter 4. Namely the **Metropolitan Life charts** and their accompanying directions on how to determine frame size, which is so vital in the proper use of their charts. Over the years the Metropolitan charts have been one of the most accepted methods to establish what a person should weigh, but as I discovered the Metropolitan charts are not the be all, end all, as they have some limitations.

Also covered in Chapter 4 is a method of what a person should weigh that is gaining favor with physicians and many in the medical community, namely the **Body Mass Index**, or **BMI**. The **BMI** does not bring weight down to an exact pound but rather indicates a general range. The **BMI** relies on the fact that people know the range where they have felt the best. From that the individual can estimate where they would probably feel the best now, and into the future.

In Chapter 4 I cover what I learned about how much food a person needs daily to maintain their present weight. After that, if you want to lose weight, reduce the calories per day and the weight comes off. That is an oversimplified statement, but it is the truth. Once the weight is off, I discovered the calories needed per day to maintain that desired weight. What I learned was surprising, to say the least. In Chapter 4 I also cover the easy way to determine your daily choleric requirement and how little I would have to cut back to maintain my desired weight. It turned out I didn't have to give up eating or starve myself to maintain my weight objective. In fact, in the end, I discovered I was now eating more, but more of the correct things.

I also learned how to determine the amount of fat in the foods I bought as well as how to find the foods that I liked that were also good for me. I need to point out that this is not a diet book. There are thousands of those out there and I am not going to repeat what they say or cover. What I am doing with this book is sharing with you what I learned in how to determine correct body weight, how many in the way of calories a person needs, and the fact we don't have to starve ourselves to maintain the optimum weight. What I have in this book is what I discovered worked in improving my general health and getting my body back in shape and extending the interval or time between the first heart attack and a follow-on event.

In Chapter 6 I learned how to determine the calories burned with the different common cardiovascular approved exercises, the likes of swimming, walking, jogging, running, etc. I discovered all I needed to know was the exercise factor for each exercise, my weight, the distance traveled, and/or time expended to determine the calories burned for each exercise.

In Chapter 7 I went into unraveling the mysteries about cholesterol tests. Essentially making sense of what cholesterol tests mean and how they affect us. By now we have all heard the words, names, and numbers bantered around like LDL's, HDL's, Triglycerides, Lipids, and the list goes on. In plain language, I try to explain what each of these terms means and how they affect us. How to understand the results of our cholesterol test.

In Chapter 8 I explain the commonsense approach to managing cholesterol. I discovered there were dozens of theories and well-meaning suggestions on how to control cholesterol, which I narrowed down to what is important, what works and what levels I could expect to realistically attain and maintain. Theoretical cholesterol goals and levels are one thing, but what is attainable, and in everyday life, is what is important.

In Chapter 9 I take on the dreaded angina. In plain language I strip away the mystery of what angina is, what are its causes and what to do when the tightness in the chest occurs. I do not downplay angina, as when it occurs it is an important indicator and is cause for concern but not cause for alarm or panic. After experiencing angina, I learned the workable measures I could take to reduce the intensity and, in some cases, prevent its occurrence altogether. That is not to say that angina is bad as it is not. Angina is a warning sign, a caution signal. If I heeded the warning, I would be fine. If I ignored the warnings, problems could occur.

Following my initial heart attack, I learned the questions I needed to ask my cardiologist. That I go into in Chapter 9. After all, this is my body and the life I am dealing with, and I needed to know what to do from this point on. I am not saying that physicians brush over what is important following the diagnosis of heart disease and a heart attack, but sometimes doctors get in a groove thinking that if the patient didn't ask a question, they must already know the answer. The physicians don't want to insult their patients or waste the patient's time discussing points he's sure the patient already knows, so passed over some things inadvertently. Wrong! But to ask those meaningful questions I had to understand what had occurred and what I needed to know to move forward. I quickly discovered the better I understood what was happening to me and had defined where I wanted to go, the better questions I could ask. After all I was dealing with my health and my future.

I made a point of making out a list of questions I had and points I needed clarified prior to visiting my physician or health care provider. This way in the heat of the visit I could make sure I covered everything that was on my mind.

Next in Chapter 10, I go into listing the most common words and phrases used in the packaging of food products. I list what I discovered, what each word meant and what were the important words to look for.

In Chapter 11 I go into how I evaluated where I was, my goals and how to set goals I could attain. Everyone needs goals, but we need goals we can hope to get to. Only then could I expect to gain the initiative and take charge of my future.

Beginning with Chapter 12 and going through Chapter 17, there are dozens of heart-healthy, low-fat recipes. There are recipes for appetizers, soups, salads, lunches, dinners, and desserts that I chose for ease of preparation; each taking just minutes to prepare with minimal kitchen skills. Along with ease of preparation, I focused on finding recipes low in fat intake. Only three of the recipes have a fat content over 9 grams with the highest being 12.3 grams, which is a little over a third of the recommended daily allowance and that is for a main course meat dish. The recipes were also chosen for their finished appearance. With a few simple suggestions, each can appear to be the work of a master chef. When it is something, people like me, who are not culinary geniuses, can whip up in a matter of minutes that is pleasant to look at as well as to the pallet.

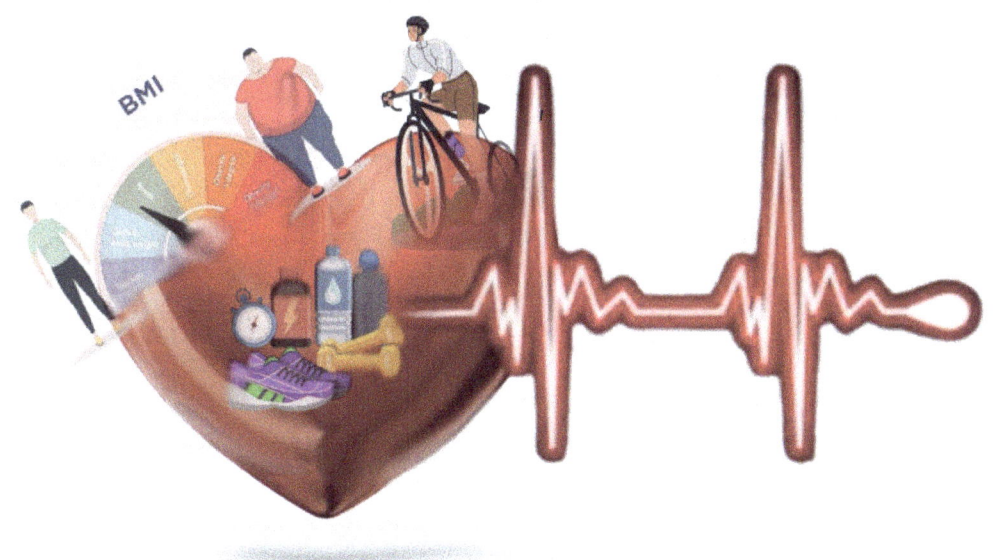

Chapter 4

How to Determine Optimum Body Weight

That is a good question, and the answer depended upon who was asked. To come up with a way to determine what I should weigh; I looked at the more widely used and generally accepted methods and charts for determining optimum body weight. Regardless of the method or chart I used, I discovered if I didn't fall right in the middle of the optimum range, it wasn't cause for concern. There was no reason for alarm. It turned out, the following widely accepted methods for determining optimum body weight were nothing more than statistical estimates. The data in the tables and charts was compiled from large population groups and while it was a good guide, it was not a hard and fast rule.

Over the years one of the most widely used weight standards has been the Metropolitan Life Insurance Tables. For years the Metropolitan Life Tables have reported weight ranges based on sex, height, and frame size. The major advantage of the Metropolitan Life charts is that they were developed by studying the weights of hundreds of thousands of people. The principal criticism of the Metropolitan Life Tables has been that their data was derived only from people capable of purchasing life insurance policies. That restricts the data to a limited segment of the general population. Second, the data was collected from each person only once, when they purchased the insurance policy. No follow-up weights were recorded. Third, the tables do not account for the person's lifestyle, occupation, or family health history.

Essentially, what the Metropolitan Life tables told me was; that of all the people who have life insurance policies who died each year, this was their height and frame size and how much they weighed when they purchased the policy, twenty, thirty, or more years before. The Metropolitan Chart is exhibit 4.1.

Metropolitan Life height and weight tables in pound

Exhibit 4.1

		WOMAN						MAN	
Height			Frame		Height			Frame	
Ft	In	Small	Medium	Large	Ft	In	Small	Medium	Large
4	10	102-111	109-121	118-131	5	2	128-134	131-141	138-150
4	11	103-113	111-123	120-134	5	3	130-136	133-143	140-153
5	0	104-115	113-126	122-137	5	4	132-136	135-145	142-156
5	1	106-118	115-129	125-140	5	5	134-140	137-148	144-160
5	2	108-121	118-132	128-143	5	6	136-142	139-151	146-164
5	3	111-124	121-135	131-147	5	7	138-145	142-154	149-168
5	4	114-127	124-138	134-151	5	8	140-148	145-157	152-172
5	5	117-130	121-141	137-155	5	9	142-151	148-160	155-176
5	6	120-133	130-144	140-159	5	10	144-154	151-163	158-180
5	7	113-136	133-147	143-163	5	11	146-157	154-166	161-184
5	8	126-139	136-150	146-170	6	0	149-160	157-170	164-188
5	9	129-142	139-153	149-170	6	1	152-164	160-174	168-192
5	10	132-145	142-156	152-170	6	2	155-168	164-184	172-197
5	11	135-148	146-159	155-176	6	3	158-172	167-182	176-202
6	0	138-151	148-162	159-179	6	4	162-176	171-187	181-207

Weights are at ages 25 to 59 based on lowest mortality.
Height includes 1" heels.

Weight for women includes 3 pounds for indoor clothing.
Weight for men includes 5 pounds for indoor clothing.

The above chart based on a weight-height mortality study conducted by the Society of Actuaries and the Association of Life Insurance Medical Directors of America, Metropolitan Life Insurance Medical Directors of America, Metropolitan life assurance Company, revised 1983

Frames Size Determination - as used by Metropolitan Life Insurance Co. in 1983
Exhibit 4.2

1. With your right arm straight down at your side, bend your forearm up a 90 degree angle to your arm.
2. Turn your palm up and point your fingers away from your body.
3. Using your thumb and index fingers of your left hand, gauge or measure the distance between the two most prominent bones on either side of your right elbow. Have a ruler handy to check the distance.
4. This is your elbow breadth.
5. Compare the measurement with the chart below for medium frame size. If your measurement is less than shown on the chart below, you have a small frame size. If your elbow bone measurement is greater than the values in the chart below, you are considered to have a large frame size.

WOMEN		MEN	
Height in 1" heels	Elbow Breadth	Height in 1" heels	Elbow Breadth
4'10" – 4'11"	2-1/4" – 2-1/2"	5'2" – 5'3"	2-1/2" – 2-7/8"
5'0" – 5'3"	2-1/4" – 2-1/2"	5'4" – 5'7"	2-5/8" – 2-7/8"
5'4" – 5'7"	2-3/8" – 2-5/8"	5'8" – 5'11"	2-3/4" – 3"
5'8" – 5'11"	2-3/8" – 2-5/8"	6'0" – 6'3"	2-3/4" – 3-1/8"
6' and over	2-1/2" – 2-3/4"	6'4" and over	2-7/8" – 3-1/4"

Metropolitan Life also put out an elaborate chart for determining frame size. It was based on the width of your elbow bone when your arm is raised at a 90-degree angle. I included that chart (exhibit 4.2) for those who want to test their measuring skills. But for those including myself who don't want to measure their elbow, there is a quicker way to determine frame size, and it does not require charts, calipers, and a ruler to measure the width of your elbow.

To determine frame size, measure the distance around the wrist with the thumb and middle finger of the opposite hand. By grasping the bony area of the wrist firmly, the object was to wrap the thumb and middle finger around my wrist.

If my thumb and middle finger just touched, I was in the middle of medium frame size.

If my thumb overlapped the middle finger slightly, I was at the lower limit of the medium frame or at the upper limit of a small frame.

If my thumb reached the first joint of the middle finger I would have had a small frame.

Conversely, if my thumb would not touch the tip of my middle finger then I was considered to have a large frame.

If the distance between my thumb and middle finger was greater than three-quarters of an inch, then I was at the upper limit of a large frame.

All I needed to do then was determine my frame size and my current height, with shoes with 1" heels, and I could use the Metropolitan Chart.

I found another method for estimating a person's desired body weight was the pound-per-inch-of-height method. According to this method, a woman should allow 100 pounds for the first five feet and then add 5 pounds for each inch above 60 inches. Based on this system a 5'6" woman should weigh 130 pounds.

100 pounds + (6" x 5 pounds) = 100 pounds + 30 pounds.

Men should start with 106 pounds for 5 feet and add 6 pounds for each inch above 60 inches. Based on this system, a 5'10' man should weigh 166 pounds.

106 pounds + (10" x 6 Pounds) = 106 pounds + 60 Pounds = 166 pounds.

The downside to this system was that it didn't take into consideration a person's frame size and general body structure. Was the person heavily muscled or lightly built? In our previous example with the 5'10" man, if he had a very heavy frame, "Large Boned" he could be on the malnourished side; and conversely, if he had a light frame, he could be overweight.

According to this method, a 6' person should weigh somewhere between 140 and 199 pounds. Not a very useful statistic.

One of the better and more popular methods in use today I discovered was what was called the Body Mass Index or **BMI**. It turned out it was currently the preferred method for determining optimum body weight. There were two ways to determine my **BMI**. Using the first way I used the mathematical formula most doctors used, which was:

Body weight in kilograms divided by the person's height in meters squared.

After I converted my bathroom scale to metric (kilograms) and my tape measured to meters I was ready to do the math. When I did the math, I came up with a number, which was the BMI. I discovered there were handy calculators for this online. When I typed the 'BMI' calculator into my computer the search engine did all the work for me.

As an alternative, I did the math and listed the results in a chart, exhibit 4.3.

BMI Exhibit 4.3 & 4.3.2 is inserted here.

So, what did the BMI tell me? The generally accepted desired BMI was between 20.0 and 25.0. According to the government, U.S.

Department of Health, etc., people with a BMI between 25.1 and 29.9 are considered overweight. People with a BMI above 30.0 are considered obese. Mortality goes up as the BMI goes up. The nice thing about the BMI, it didn't narrow my weight range down to a tight little box. If I came up with a number between 20.0 and 25.0 that was considered normal.

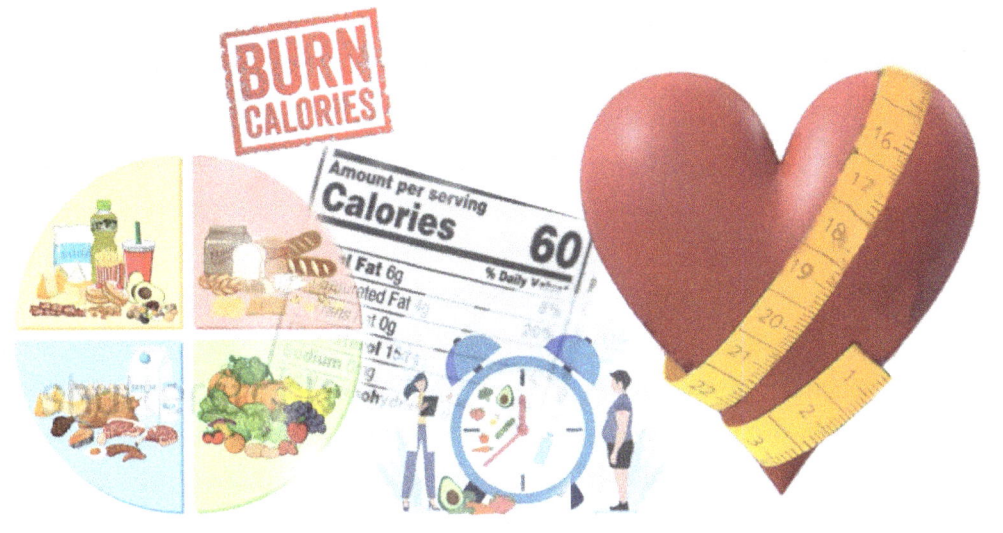

Chapter 5

Food – How much do I need?

How much do I have to cut back to lose weight?

What do I have to do to get to my desired weight?

In the past most books have referred to this process of losing weight as "*your diet*". Unfortunately, the word '*Diet*' has taken on the strong secondary meaning of the process of 'attempting to lose weight' or the practice of 'food deprivation – starving' to lose weight. Whereas in reality, 'diet' really means the normal amount and types of food and drink consumed for healthy sustenance.

That brings up two major questions:

A. How much should I cut back on to lose weight?

B. Once I have lost weight and reached my desired goal, how much food can I eat to maintain my optimal weight where I neither gained, nor lost weight?

There were several ways of determining this. One way was to calculate 'Basal Metabolism'. Add to that an amount for 'Physical Activity' and the 'Thermic effect associated with the consumption of food' and I came up with total *energy* used. Sounds complicated, well it was.

Another way was to use the Harris-Benedict equation to determine 'Basal Metabolism' which does not take into consideration 'Physical Activity' and the 'Thermic Effect' resulting from the energy the body expends in consuming and processing what I eat.

A third way to calculate the average calories I could consume in a day; where I neither gained nor lost weight, and produced results comparable to those derived by the above two methods was from a book titled, 'Health and Fitness Through Physical Activity', by Michael L. Pollock, Jack H. Wilmore, and Samuel M. Fox III, published by John Wiley & Sons:

A. For a normal, healthy adult, the book's authors said to multiply body weight by one of the following factors to determine the average number of calories consumed or burned in 24 hours. The factors listed below apply for either men or women. The activity levels are somewhat open for interpretation, but each activity level takes into consideration the normal non-work-a-day activities.

Mostly sedentary activity: (mostly sitting, no exercise);	15.5
Light activity: (less sitting, some walking):	19.2
Moderately active: (a store clerk, a teacher):	20.4
Heavy activity: (construction work, etc.):	22.8

Therefore, if I were a person working in an office who walked a block to the bus, rode it to work, walked a block to my job from the bus stop, sat all day, and repeated the process getting home, and then sat watching TV until bedtime; I would have been classified as a person having a 'Sedentary' lifestyle. As an example, if I weighed 163 pounds, multiply that times the 15.5 factor, and then my calorie needs would be: 163 x 15.5 = 2526 calories for the 24-hour day.

Likewise, if the 163-pound person above were relatively active, such as a clerk in a warehouse-type store did a fair amount of walking and standing each day, and weighed 163 pounds, the calorie factor multiplier would be 20.4. That person's calorie requirements for the day would then be:

163 x 20.4 = 3,325 calories in 24 hours.

One thing to note, these calorie calculations were strictly estimates of what a person under the age of 30 would consume in 24 hours, but it was at least a place to start. It was stated that 100 calories per day should be deducted for every 10 years a person was over 30. Otherwise, if the person is 39 or less, deduct 100 calories per day. If the person is 49 or less, deduct 200 calories per day. If the person was under 59 deduct 300 calories per day. For people over 60 deduct 400 calories per day. The exceptions to this adjustment were mothers who were breastfeeding. Likewise, teenagers and young children all require more calories. I learned that for those people who are interested in finding out their caloric daily requirement, they need to contact a registered dietitian.

B. How to lose weight. To lose one pound per week our 163-pound person would need to burn 3500 more calories per week than they ate. A bit simplified, but 3500 calories roughly equal one pound. Therefore, from the example above, the 163 pounds, moderately active 52-year-old person's normal calorie requirements per day would be 3325 calories, minus 300 calories because the person was over 30, (100 calories for each

10 years over 30) for a net projected 3025 calorie requirement per day. That 3025 times the 7 days in a week mean that person would require 21,175 calories per week to maintain their weight where they neither gained nor lost weight. For that person to lose two pounds per week, that person would need to deduct 2 x 3500 calories or 7000 calories per week from their caloric intake to lose two pounds per week.

The math was simple: 21,175 calories minus 7,000 calories = 14,175 caloric consumption per week. 14,175 divided by seven days = 2,025 calories per day. So, if that 52-year-old, 163-pound person wanted to lose two pounds per week they would need to reduce their daily caloric intake to 2,025 calories per day or less.

Another example is a 175-pound person with a sedentary lifestyle who is 45 years old, their normal daily caloric requirement to maintain that weight would be: 175 pounds times 15.5 multiplier factor = 2,712 calories less 200 calories per day because they are over 30 and under 50 years old would equal a daily caloric maintenance requirement of 2,512 calories per day. That number times the seven days in a week and the person was eating 17,584 calories per week. To lose the two pounds per week the person would have to reduce their food intake (calorie intake) per week by 7,000 calories. Therefore, to lose the two pounds per week, they would deduct 7,000 calories from 17,584 for 10, 584 which equals the total weekly allotment and that divided by seven days means the person would need to eat 1,512calories or less per day to lose two pounds per week.

I learned that when I was working to lose the 40 plus pounds that weighing each morning and maintaining a record was important. I made a point to weigh myself at the same time, right after I got up each day. While on the diet I wanted to see the needle on the scale creep lower and each morning, and it did. If on the off chance one week I wasn't weight at the previous rate, I would sit down and list what I was eating that I shouldn't to keep on my weight reduction program.

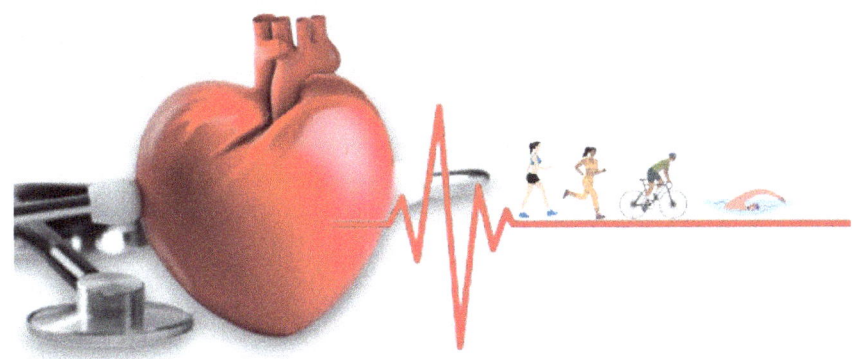

Chapter 6

Activity Calorie Consumption Easy Calculation

There are literally hundreds of different activities a person can participate in from Archery to Zumba and they all burn calories. To list all the possible activities and their associated variables and then the methods for calculating the calories burned would require another book double this size. Even at that, it would only touch the subject. Not to mention, it would be enormously technical. Likewise, there are any number of devices available that a person can wear on their body that will keep track of steps taken, heart rate, calories burned, and on and on.

What I am going to write about is how I learned to estimate calories burned for several generally accepted cardiovascular activities, or exercises, without using some device you can strap on your wrist or around the waist, or on your leg.

As a result, I focused on activities that have the least variables, namely the endurance ones, walking, running, swimming, jogging, and bicycling. These are activities that can be done with or without a partner and are activities where both the duration (time) and intensity are controllable. Because these activities bring our heart rate up to the plateau (steady rate) and the rate (beats per minute) remains relatively constant throughout the time we are doing the exercise, it is considered a cardiovascular exercise. Also, these cardiovascular exercises can be performed daily at a predictable level of intensity.

The formula for calculating the approximate calories an adult person would burn to do any of these exercises is as follows:

Multiply Your Weight (YW) times the Activity Factor (AF) for a particular activity times the Distance (D) or duration. If we type in Activity Factor and search online, we'll be presented with dozens of studies that list activity factors for 'Sedentary', 'Light Activity', 'Moderate Activity', 'Very Active', and 'Extremely Active'. Fine, but how do those factors correspond to 'Walking', 'Jogging', 'Running' etcetera? The more I studied the more I felt there had to be a way to calculate Calories burned doing Specific Activities. Using the Activity Factors I found in the previously referenced book, 'Health and Fitness Through Physical Activity' I found a simple way to determine the calories burned doing routine cardiovascular exercises.

Example - Jogging: A 173-pound person jogs three miles a day on relatively flat pavement and wants to know the approximate calories burned doing that exercise.

The Activity Factor (AF) for jogging is: .89 calories per mile of (D) Distance for every Pound of the person's weight (BW).

This can be written: Jogging AF = .89 cal/ml/lb of BW

The calorie calculation works as follows:

Calories Burned (CB) = (AF) x (BW) x (D)

Therefore: CB = (.89) x (173) pounds x (3) miles = 462 calories burned.

It must be noted the calories burned in the example above are approximate as there are more influencing factors other than just weight and speed on calorie consumption. Jogging or walking in a stiff head wind burns more calories than walking or jogging with the wind. Walking, jogging, or running on a cold day also increases the calories burned as does doing likewise on a very hot day. Rugged, hilly terrain will also increase the calories burned as opposed to that on a smooth, level track. Therefore, the results derived using these calculation methods will produce a close approximation idea or estimate of calorie consumption per each type of activity.

Walking

The (AF) Activity Factor for walking averages out to around .72 calories/mile/pound of Body Weight, whether it be at two miles per hour or the recommended target speed for a vigorous cardiovascular workout of four miles per hour.

In my case when I got down to 185 pounds and was walking six miles each morning, rain or shine, uphill or down, 365 days per year, I was burning 799.2 calories, or rounded off 800 calories per day, which equated to a little over a pound a week.

CB – calories burned = (.72) x (185) x (6) = 800 Calories burned.

Note: The calculated calories burned are approximate as there are more influencing factors other than just your weight and speed on calorie consumption.

Walking into a stiff headwind I burned considerably more calories than walking with the wind. Walking on a cold day also increases calorie consumption, as did walking on a very hot day. Rugged, hilly terrain will also increase the calories burned as opposed to a smooth-level track.

Therefore, the results computed using these methods will give us a close approximation of calorie consumption per type of activity.

Jogging

The (AF) Activity Factor for all forms or speeds of jogging averages out to around .89 cal/mi/lb of **Your Weight.**

Otherwise, a 158-pound person jogging two miles burns 281 calories.

Calories Burned = (.89) x (158) x (2) = 281 calories

Note: Speed of jogging does not really affect the calories burned. The calories burned equates to the amount of energy required to propel our body in a jogging motion. The same was true with walking. There again, the only factor speed plays is the length of time it takes to cover a set distance.

Running

The **(AF)** Activity Factor for running outdoors on a varied terrain is nearly the same as for jogging at .89. Some studies put the **Activity**

Factor a little lower, at around .86 Cal/mi/lb of **Your Weight** for running on a uniform track, whether it be indoors or out.

Which works out: A 194-pound person running 2-1/2 miles on an indoor track burns approximately 417 calories.

Calories Burned = (AF .86) x (194 lb) x (2.5 mi) = 417 calories burned.

Running on a treadmill; is frequently referred to as running in place.

Because the motor driving the belt is moving the running surface past the person, whereby the person's leg muscles are involved only in moving the person's legs and feet and not the whole body, the **(AF) Activity Factor** is roughly half the number used for running on a physical track or: .43 Cal/mi/lb of **Your**

Weight.

Written as: 205-pound person running five miles on a treadmill burns approximately 441 calories.

Calories Burned = (AF .43) x (205 lb) x (5 mi) = 441 calories burned.

Bicycling

The (AF) Activity Factor for working out on an indoor or stationary bicycle averages out at .25 cal/mi/lb of Your Weight. The same cannot be said for bicycling outdoors. If you are in Florida on relatively flat ground riding a single-speed bike, then probably yes, the Activity Factor or .25 will probably apply. But most areas are not as uniformly level as Florida and people use multi-speed bicycles which makes calculating calories burned nearly impossible. Therefore, you will have to judge your own situation, but for the moment we will say the bicycling Activity Factor of .25 is for stationary bicycling.

Example: A 240-pound person pedaling eight miles on a stationary bicycle burns approximately 480 calories.

Calories Burned = (AF .25) x (240 lb) x (8 mi) = 480 Calories Burned.

Swimming

The **(AF) A**ctivity **F**actor for swimming is based on hundred foot pool lengths at: .039 cal/100 feet/lb of **Y**our **W**eight. A little math is required to convert laps in the pool to distance in feet covered.

Example: A 160-pound person swimming 25 laps in a 50 meter pool (50 meters = 164 feet) burns 512 calories.

25 laps = 50 lengths and 50 lengths x 164 feet = 8,200 feet or 82/100's

Calories burned = (AF .039) x (160 lb) x (82/100's) = 512 calories burned.

Remember back in Chapter 5, "to lose one pound a person needs to burn 3500 more calories than they take in".

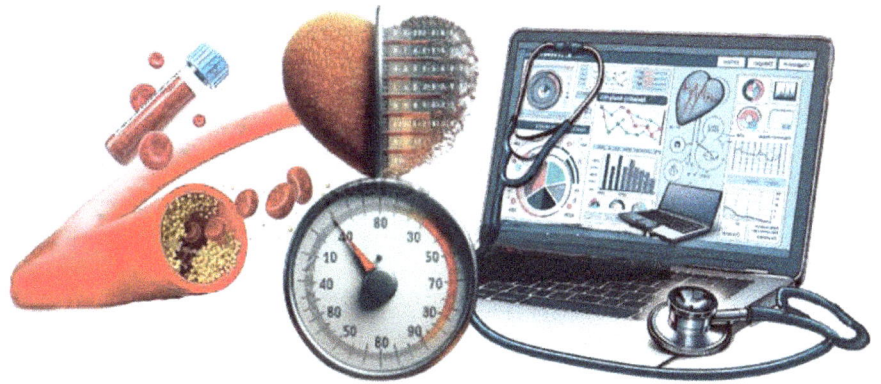

Chapter 7

Making sense of your Cholesterol test results

We've all seen those numbers for LDL and HDL and Triglycerides and the total cholesterol number. Some physicians go to the trouble to explain their meaning, but the majority of doctors will just say 'Your cholesterol is too high, and you need this medication or that. And you ask, "How long will I be on this medication?" and the physician's common response, "forever." So, if a person is going to be with this forever, it is only right to understand what each term means.

Cholesterol (ko-Les-te-rol): A waxy lipid or fatty structure. There are 18 different types of cholesterol and other fats in our blood and not all of them are bad. To put the record straight, there is cholesterol in every cell in our bodies. Certain levels of cholesterol are required for normal living. But exceed the 'normal' levels and there's trouble. Excessive levels are the problem as the extra fat or cholesterol unfortunately can adhere to the walls of our arteries and veins which can restrict the normal flow of blood and therefore increase the risk of a heart attack or stroke.

LDL Cholesterol: Low Density Lipoprotein. This is the cholesterol needed to build and replace cells in our body but in excess, LDL cholesterol is harmful and is considered the bad cholesterol when there is too much of it in our blood and the extra LDL adheres to the walls of our arteries and restricts the flow of blood. This is the cholesterol we must maintain within balanced levels and if the level of LDL gets elevated, it needs to be brought back in balance.

HDL Cholesterol: High Density Lipoprotein. This is the healthy or good cholesterol. This is the cholesterol we must raise if it is low. HDL works to pick up LDL and transport the excess LDL back to the liver for reprocessing and excretion; thereby reducing the LDL level.

Triglycerides (try-GLISS-uh-ride): The most common form of lipids or fat in our bodies and our food. Triglycerides are present in the blood to enable bidirectional transference of adipose fat and blood glucose from the liver, and are a major component of human skin cells.

The Mayo Clinic summarized triglycerides and cholesterol lipids in an article they posted on line https://www.mayoclinic.org/diseases-conditions/high-blood-cholesterol/in-depth%20/%20triglycerides/art-20048186. Specifically, they stated "Triglycerides and cholesterol are separate types of lipids that circulate in your blood. Triglycerides store unused calories and provide your body with energy, and cholesterol is used to build cells and certain hormones. Because triglycerides and cholesterol can't dissolve in blood, they circulate throughout your body with the help of proteins that transport the lipids (lipoproteins)."

The National Cholesterol Education Program has set the following levels for triglyceride levels.

Level	Interpretation
Less that 150 mg/dl	Normal range – low risk
150 - 199 mg/dl	Slightly above normal
200 - 499 mg/dl	Some risk
500 or higher	Vary high - high risk

These levels are tested after fasting 8 to 12 hours.

Triglyceride levels remain temporarily high for a period after eating.

The American Heart Association recommends an optimal triglyceride level less than 100 mg/dl to improve heart health.

The Cholesterol Blood Test:

When the doctor orders a "***Cholesterol Blood Test***" what he is really requesting is a ***Lipid Panel***. The patient is instructed to fast (abstain from eating or drinking anything but water) for 10 to 12 hours prior to having a blood sample drawn at the laboratory. It is most convenient to schedule the lab appointment for the first thing in the morning. Done that way the test is the least disruptive. The patient is instructed not to eat anything after 6:00 pm the evening before.

Understanding the Test Results:

The results of the Lipid Panel test take about 24 to get back from the laboratory. The results will be listed as: Total Blood Cholesterol Level, the LDL Level, the HDL level and the Triglyceride level. The results will be listed in mg/dl which stands for milligrams per deciliter (deciliter = 1/10 of a liter). Listed below are the generally accepted risk ranges.

The 'Low Risk' ranges are what the physician will encourage the patient to attain.

The 'Borderline High Risk' range is just that. Not cause for alarm but will deserve close following. The physician will possibly even suggest ways to bring the level lower.

The 'High Risk' range is exactly that. The values in this range are real attention getters. If the patient is in the 'High Risk' range on all values, the physician usually requires immediate examination, evaluation and alteration of the patient's eating habits. The physician might even say, "to reduce the risk of future heart attacks the patient will have to get the bad cholesterol levels down."

Total Blood Cholesterol Levels:

Low Risk - LESSS THAN 200 MG/DL

Borderline High Risk - 200 mg/dl to 239 mg/dl

High Risk - 240 mg/dl and higher

LDL Cholesterol Levels:

Low Risk - Less than 130 mg/dl

Borderline High Risk - 130 mg/dl to 159 mg/dl

High Risk - 160 mg/dl and above.

Note: If the patient has had a heart attack the goal is to lower the LDL level to or below 100 mg/dl if possible.

Triglyceride Cholesterol Levels:

Low Risk - Less than 200 mg/dl

Borderline High Risk - 200 mg/dl to 400 mg/dl

High Risk - 400 mg/dl to 1000 mg/dl

Very High Risk - Over 1000 mg/dl

HDL Cholesterol Levels:

There are no set ranges for HDL levels, rather HDL is used in calculating a ratio between Total Cholesterol to HDL. The ratio is determined by dividing **Total Cholesterol** by **HDL**. The result is a ratio. Example: If Total Cholesterol at 200 mg/dl and HDL is 50 mg/dl the ratio would be four to one, or 4:1 Likewise if Total Cholesterol was 125 mg/dl and HDL was 39 the ratio would be 3.2 to one or 3.2:1.

Optimum Range - 3:1 to 3.5:1

Desirable Range - 3.5:1 to 4:1

Borderline Range - 4.1:1 to 5:1

Undesirable Range - 5.2 and higher.

If the patient's ratio is in the 4.1: to 5:1 area that indicates that the HDL or 'Good' Cholesterol is too low, or the Total Cholesterol level is too high. The physician will advise the patient to reduce their intake of fatty foods and possibly increase their exercise levels. One of the main benefits of exercise is that even as little as 30 minutes a day of brisk walking can increase HDL levels by upwards of 10% or more.

Managing cholesterol levels is essential to reduce the incidence of heart attacks and strokes.

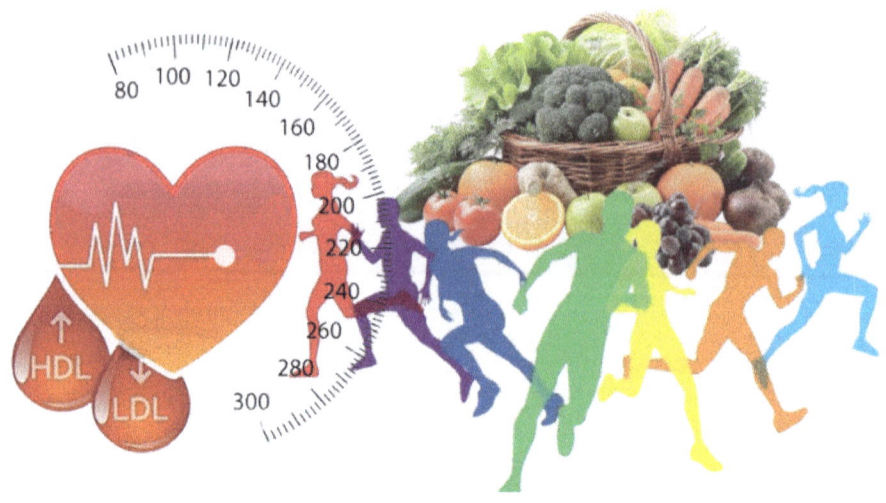

Chapter 8

A commonsense approach to Cholesterol management

Just because the LDL and Triglyceride levels are too high, and the HDL level is too low, and the Ratio between Total Cholesterol and HDL is too high, there is no reason to panic. Some measures can be taken to remedy the situation.

When the physician says the cholesterol levels must come down, what the doctor is saying is that the intake of fatty foods, primarily foods with saturated fats found in animal and dairy products such as beef, lamb, pork, cheese, butter, lard, whole milk, and cream, as well as some plant-based oils such as palm oil, palm kernel oil, and coconut oil needs to be reduced. The physician is not saying for the patient to eliminate them all altogether but to monitor the amount of saturated fat we eat and where possible limit consumption as much as possible. But as said before, not all cholesterol is bad, just most of it when consumed in excess.

What the physician wants, is for the patient to work to elevate or increase the consumption of HDL's (High-Density Lipoprotein) Cholesterol while at the same time reducing the overall fat in the diet, primarily reducing the consumption of foods high in saturated fats. Unfortunately, foods high in HDL are not something that can be shopped for. The 'Nutrition Facts' label on every food in the store does not contain one word about HDL content. So where do people get HDL? The truth is, that the body produces HDL. HDL is produced by the liver and small intestines. The objective is to increase the production of HDL while at the same time reducing the LDL.

There are several ways we can increase HDL levels. One way is exercise. Exercising at least 45 minutes a day, four times a week will go far to increase HDL. While 30 minutes of brisk walking three times a week is the minimum, per the American Heart Association, 45 minutes four times a week is recommended. Regular exercise is the easiest and fastest way to raise HDL levels. Regular exercise is known to raise HDL levels by as much as 5 mg/dl.

Next, lose weight. Shedding the extra pounds will go far in increasing the HDL levels. Getting down to a BMI (Body Mass Index) of 22 to 24 will do much toward increasing the HDL level as well. Another thing a patient can do to increase HDL levels is if they smoke, STOP. 'Quit Smoking'. In my case before my heart attack, I smoked 3 packs a day. I know that was ridiculous. I had to stop! Not smoking would assist in elevating my HDL level as would eating three meals a day, regular exercising, and weight control. I learned that only focusing on one of the above lifestyle changes by itself would not have the same effect as doing all of the above together; namely, exercising, controlling my weight, not smoking, and eating regular balanced meals a day.

After addressing HDL, the focus must be on controlling LDL Cholesterol. To this end, the lifestyle changes taken to increase the HDL levels are the same as those to reduce LDL Cholesterol levels. Increasing the HDL levels is a start. While medication is one approach to reduce LDL levels, physicians will agree it should never be the first line of defense, most doctors will agree using medications to control LDL levels is a last resort. The truth is, there is no magic pill or medicine out there that a person can take to lower LDL levels while at the same time continuing to consume foods high in saturated fats and cholesterol while living a sedentary lifestyle. The bottom line, people with high Cholesterol will need to take charge of their health. They will have to watch what they eat, and reduce consuming saturated fats while increasing their activity (exercising, i.e. walking, jogging, running, swimming, etc).

Only after patients make a genuine effort to bring their cholesterol levels down using diet, exercise, and weight management, will physicians resort to prescribing medication, keeping in mind all medications come with a lengthy list of side effects. Many of those side effects are far worse than the condition that we are attempting to remedy.

The first and foremost important step that I could take to take control of the cholesterol in my body was to reduce the consumption of saturated fats. Excessive consumption of 'Saturated Fats' was in my case, as it is in most cases, the main contributing factor to elevated cholesterol. The American Institute of Health and The American Heart Association have gone so far as to recommend that people seeking a healthier life, need to consume less than 20 grams of saturated fat per day. Some groups have gone so far as to recommend limiting daily consumption of saturated fat to less than 15 grams per day total fat consumption to less than 65 grams per day, and cholesterol to less than 300 milligrams per day.

To do that for the first few weeks out of the hospital and making a concerted effort to live healthier, I jotted down the saturated fats I consumed as well as the total fat and cholesterol I consumed. At first, it was a bit of a chore, but in no time, it became second nature as I became familiar with what I could eat and what foods I needed to avoid. It wasn't long and I became very conscious of the contents of the foods I ate. By keeping track of the Total Fat and Cholesterol in the different foods, I could shop for those healthier items and avoid the fat-laden ones. One of the things I learned up front was that eating healthy, namely foods low in fat, not only were they very filling, but they were also tasty and nourishing. It turns out the food industry has made significant progress in lowering the fat content in their products while maintaining flavor. If you haven't shopped for 'reduced fat', and 'low fat' or 'fat-free' foods lately you might be as amazed as I was as to what is out there and how good it tastes. After a while, I was able to calculate the allowed 'saturated fat', 'total fat', and 'cholesterol' levels without using a paper. I quickly got a feel for what I could eat and what I shouldn't. I knew what to do if I were with friends and was served a fast-food greasy burger and fries or a thick crust pan pizza, I would eat the burger without the bun and scrape off the topping on the pizza and eat that by itself. For the next few days, I watched what I ate and made sure to avoid as much saturated fatty foods as possible.

If I were on the road and had a choice when I got hungry for lunch, rather than whip through a drive-through window and get a greasy burger and fries like I used to do, I sought out a 'Subway' or the like and had something just about as quick, and far better for me.

I discovered the secondary benefit of watching daily fat intake. Not only was the low-fat diet good for the heart and the blood flowing through my system but getting the fat and cholesterol levels down was working wonders with my weight reduction program. By doing that and walking my 6 miles every morning, I went from 232 pounds to 182 pounds in 6 months. That's right, I lost 50 pounds in 6 months and never looked back.

To help in making sense of the allowable fats, cholesterol, sodium, potassium, carbohydrates, dietary fiber, and protein allowed daily, I have listed the recommended amounts for a 2000-calorie-a-day diet. The 2000 calorie-a-day diet was the amount my physician said I should stay at, considering I had been diagnosed with coronary heart disease (CHD). For others, who are smaller or larger the physician would probably recommend different calorie amounts.

Like it or not, my CAD was not about to go away. As my doctor said, when managed properly, coronary artery disease is easy to live with. As he said, because I was in a heart attack risk group I needed to stay with the lower values listed on the 'Nutrition Facts' labels on each food package. I asked if the 'Nutrition Facts' listed were specific for male or female, young or old and his nutritionist said it was a good guide for everyone. She said staying with the 2000 calorie-a-day dietary allowances for fats, etc. was just a good guide. Below is the chart she gave me.

		Calories per Day	
		2000	2000
Total Fat	Less than	65g	80g
Saturated Fat	Less than	20g	25g
Cholesterol	Less than	300mg	300mg
Sodium (salt)	Less than	2,400mg	2,400mg
Potassium	Less than	3,000mg	3,000mg
Total Carbohydrate		300g	375g
Dietary Fiber		25g	30g
Protein		50g	65g

g = gram   mg = milligram

Calories per gram:

Each gram of Fat	equals 9 calories
Each gram of Carbohydrate	equals 4 calories
Each gram of Protein	equals 4 calories

The nutritionist also stated that because I had had a heart attack and was diagnosed with coronary artery disease, and therefore my doctor was concerned about monitoring my blood pressure, she said a low sodium diet was vital. By low sodium diet, she meant take the salt shaker off the dinner table. She stated that under normal dietary conditions all the salt I would need was already in the foods I ate. I did not need to add salt to my meal. She pointed out that 'Salt' was an acquired taste. She said to go without adding salt to my food for a month and I would discover that I could eliminate adding salt to everything I ate. She also pointed out that many of the foods I had been accustomed to automatically shook on more salt, what I tasted when I ate scrambled eggs or cottage cheese was salt. So, I did what she said. I hid the saltshaker for a month and there it remained.

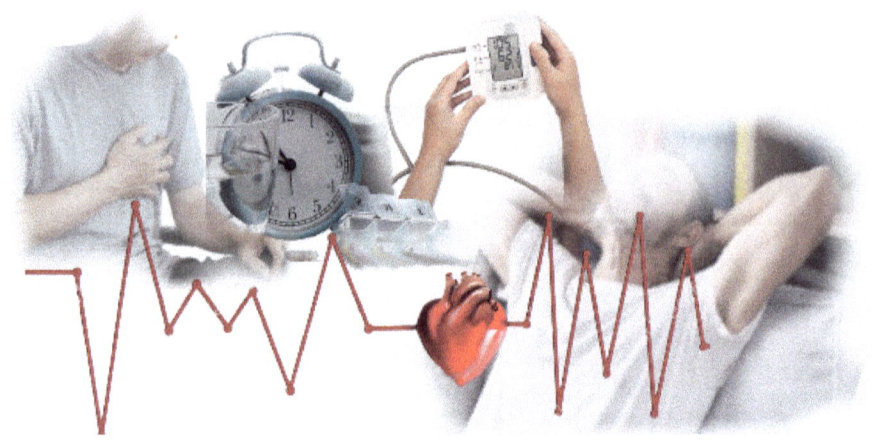

Chapter 9

Understanding Angina

W e've all heard the word, Angina, what is it? Is it a life threatening sentence? Does it mean we are at death's door? Does it mean we are about to be buried? On the contrary. Turns out, Angina is the chest pain or discomfort that occurs when the heart muscles do not get enough oxygen. Really? When I first heard that I blinked. That to me sounded like a heart attack. When I studied Angina, I came to realize it really wasn't a heart attack. In fact, there is a distinct difference.

A heart attack occurs when the blood flow to a part of the heart muscle is suddenly cut off by a major blockage in an artery and that in turn produces a severe uninterrupted pain in the center of the chest.

Which is exactly what I experienced with my first heart attack. I needed help and I needed it right then. The medic one unit could not get to my house fast enough. I was sure I was going to die. The pain alone made me feel that way. As it turned out the Medic One unit got there in time and got me to the hospital and the rest I have already covered.

With Angina, the flow of blood to the heart muscle is restricted, not cut off. By restricted, it means blood is getting to the heart muscles that work to pump the blood around the system, it's just that the heart is not getting enough blood to allow it, (the heart) to pump at 100%. Angina occurs when the heart is unable to pump at the capacity of what the body needs. My doctor pointed out that this was like when a person runs up a flight of stairs or climbs a steep hill and gets out of breath. Following that the body and muscles are demanding more oxygen than the lungs and blood can supply. In an out of breath situation when the person stops and rests briefly, the shortness of breath quickly disappears. He said the same is true with an angina attack. The tightness or chest discomfort I would feel is an indicator that the muscles of the heart are not getting as much oxygen as my activity level is demanding.

I learned that Angina, like a heart attack most frequently occurs during above-average levels of physical exertion or periods of high emotional stress. The tightness discomfort or pain in the chest experienced is a warning sign. To begin with, it is telling me, the recovered heart attack victim; to stop doing what I was doing that caused the angina discomfort in the first place. If after a few minutes, the discomfort does not go away I am to take one of the nitroglycerin tablets my doctor prescribed. He instructed me to slip it under my tongue, sit back, and try to relax. If after five minutes the discomfort persists, I am to place a second tablet under my tongue. I am going to wait another five minutes and if the pain is still there, I am to take a third tablet. He said 3 tablets in 15 minutes was the maximum dosage. If the third tablet does not relieve the pain or discomfort, the problem is more severe than a minor angina attack. He said if 911 was not available where I was at, I needed to get someone to take me to a hospital emergency room. I am not to call him and see if that is what he wants me to do. I am to get to the hospital first. The hospital will contact my doctor upon my admission.

My doctor pointed out that the above three tablets and a quick trip to the ER are the exception rather than the rule. He stated, that in most Angina situations, just stopping the activity will be sufficient to cause the discomfort and pain to pass. If after the discomfort passes, I am cleared to try the activity again, but at a lower intensity. If I do and Angina doesn't reoccur then I have learned my limit.

Other signs the physician needs to know about are:

If Angina reoccurs with lesser amounts of exertion for that activity.

If the Angina lasts longer and is more severe each time it occurs.

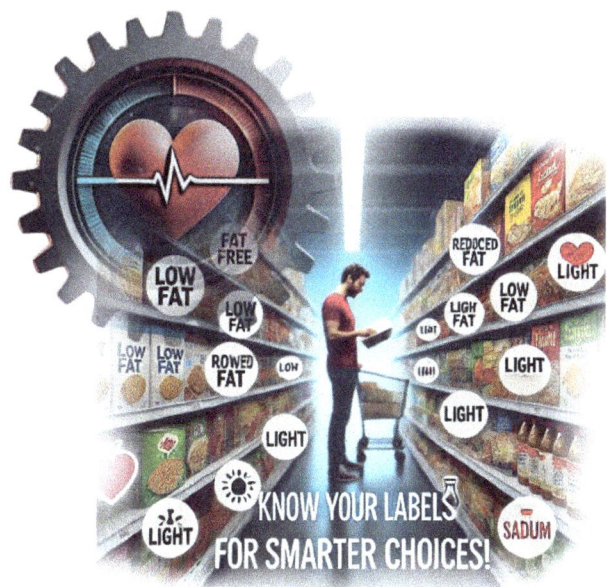

Chapter 10

Food packaging key words and what they mean.

Anutritionist I met with said when I am in the store I should look for the following key words; 'Fat Free', 'Low Fat', 'Reduced Fat', 'Cholesterol Free', 'Low in Cholesterol', 'Reduced Cholesterol', and 'Light', or 'Lite'. Armed with those I should be able to navigate the mine field of package labeling.

Key Word	What the 'Key Word' means.
Fat Free	Less than 0.5 grams of fat per serving.
Low Fat	Less than 3 grams of fat per serving

Reduced Fat/Less Fat	At least 25% less fat per serving than the regular version.
Lean	Less than 10 grams of fat, 4 grams of saturated fat and less than 95 milligrams of cholesterol.
Extra Lean	Less than 5 grams of fat, 2 grams of saturated fat and 95 milligrams of cholesterol per serving.
Low in saturated Fat	Less than 1 gram of saturated fat per serving and not more than 15% of calories from saturated fatty acids.
Low Cholesterol	Less than 20 milligrams of cholesterol and less than 2 grams of saturated fat per serving.
Reduced Cholesterol	25% or less cholesterol than the higher regular version and less than 2 grams of saturated fat per serving.
Calorie Free	Less than 5 calories per serving.
Light (Lite)	1/3 less calories or no more than 1/2 the fat of the regular higher calorie, higher fat version, and no more than 1/2 of the sodium of the higher sodium version.
Sugar Free	Less than 0.5 grams of sugar per serving.
Sodium Free	Less than 5 milligrams of sodium per serving and no sodium chloride (NACL) in the product.
Very Low Sodium	Less than 35 milligrams of sodium per serving.
Low Sodium	Less than 140 milligrams of sodium per serving.
Reduced or Less Sodium	25% or more less sodium per serving than the regular version.
High Fiber	5 grams or more fiber per serving.
Good Source of Fiber	Good Source of Fiber

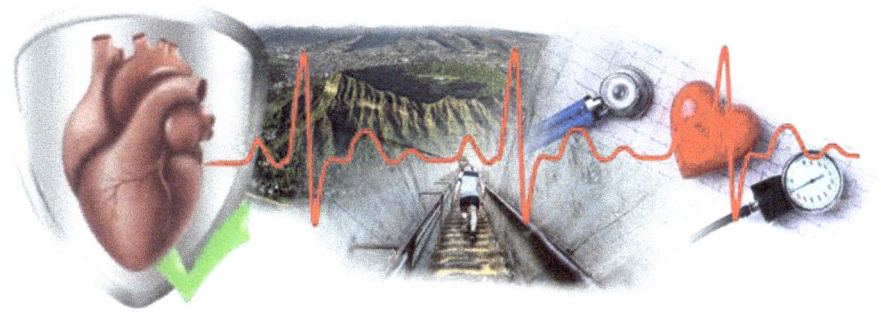

Chapter 11

16 Years Later - the Second Time Around

The first 9 chapters, plus the recipe section at the end of this book was what I wrote a year or so following my first heart attack. At that time, I thought I had all the answers. I had survived a major medical event, a heart attack. I was still alive. I had two stents in my heart. My blood was once again flowing freely. My heart was pumping like it should. I was walking 6 miles a day and enjoying it.

Following that initial heart attack, I made it my goal to do everything in my power to never have another. One heart attack was enough. It was painful . . . extremely so. It was frightening. That's right, it was very scary. For a brief time, I thought I was going to die. It was something I did not want to experience again. Toward that goal of preventing a future heart attack, I watched my diet. I focused on fat-free and low-fat meals with minimal amounts of cholesterol and saturated fats. I monitored my caloric intake. I exercised faithfully. I shed 50 pounds. I went from 232 pounds to 182 pounds. Not only did I lose that much weight; by exercising, watching what I ate and the amount, I kept the 50 pounds off.

In the process of working toward that goal of no future heart attacks, I exercised faithfully. I walked daily. Every day of the year. A solid 6 miles each day, rain or shine, snow or blazing hot. I would leave my house shortly after 6 AM each morning and set out on my 6 + mile walking adventure. I had a half dozen different routes I would take but they all were the minimum of 6 miles each. On especially nice days in the summer, when it wasn't too hot, I would walk 9 miles. I would pick my days in June, July and August.

I did take out six weeks from walking one winter when on my way back and less than 100 yards from my house I slipped on an icy patch and fell. I broke the two bones in my right arm, just above my wrist. Fortunately, my youngest daughter was home, and she took me to the emergency room. An hour or so later I was back home with a plaster cast from my fingertips to above my elbow. I could not flex my arm. I also came home with a set of instructions, (**orders from the doctor**) not to walk for the next six weeks; or until after the cast was off. The orthopedic physician did not want to see me again with the other wrist fractured. And neither did I for that matter, so I followed what he said.

A couple of years later I went to Hawaii on business, specifically Honolulu and Pearl Harbor. While there I took out a day to do a little sightseeing. One of the attractions I visited was Diamond Head, the 760-foot-tall extinct volcano, along Oahu's south shore. While at Diamond Head Park I could not resist doing the walk to the observation lookout area at the top, with the 360-degree view of the island. Upon on arrival there you can purchase a tee shirt that states you did the 100 stairs walk at Diamond Head, and I did, and I have worn the shirt proudly. Unlike a lot of people younger than me, I made the 100 steps to the top without stopping to rest or catch my breath. I had recovered from my heart attack. I was mended.

I continued my walking and following my low-fat diet program and was going along quite comfortably. The fact that I had a history of cardiovascular disease was something I was aware of but didn't dwell on, until 16 plus years after that first attack, while rebuilding a fence gate, I felt tightness in my chest, a dull pain. It was strenuous work, but I felt I was up to it. I didn't give it a thought that I might be pushing myself. As I was wrestling the wooden gate into position the tightness in my chest grew. It became a noticeable pain. I knew it wasn't a heart attack, as the pain was not that severe. But it was a pain and not just a heavy feeling in my chest. What immediately came to mind was this angina thing, or maybe it was heartburn, because of something I had recently eaten for lunch. Upon completion of the work on the wooden gate, I drove a mile or so to my house. Once there I took a couple of antacids and laid down for a few minutes. To my relief, the discomfort subsided, and a half hour later was gone. Satisfied with the pain in my chest had not been angina, but heartburn I continued with my day. A few days later, while not doing any strenuous exercise or work, the tightness in my chest reoccurred. At first, when that happened, I would stretch out, take a couple of antacids and the discomfort would subside and eventually disappear. A few days later when the tightness in my chest would not go away, I told my wife, and she thought it best she takes me to the emergency room just to be on the safe side. Upon being admitted to the ER I told the nurse what I had been experiencing and she brought in the cardiologist on call. The cardiologist listened to me describe my experience and thought it best to do an MRI. Upon completion of the test, he said there was an indication there was some abnormality with my heart that warranted further evaluation and admitted me to the hospital for the night.

After a few more tests, the cardiologist concluded I had had a heart attack, all be it mild, and my original cardiologist, who installed the 2 stents sixteen and a half years before, was called in. He reviewed the tests and told me the 2 stents needed to be replaced. He pointed out that considering the average useful expectancy of stents was six to seven years, and that my stents had been in for sixteen and a half years, they needed to be replaced. A day later, he proceeded. Rather than go through an artery in my groin, as he had done sixteen and a half years before, he said he would pop into an artery just above my wrist and run his probe to my heart from there. He said he would be giving me a mild general anesthetic to ease any anxiety I might have and that I would feel nothing, and the procedure would be all over in a matter of minutes. Remembering my previous reaction to a mild general anesthetic, I said I wanted the procedure done with a local anesthetic. He balked at that until I reminded him of the past reaction I had had to general anesthetic. To that, he said "Okay," he would do it under local anesthetic but at the first indication I was getting stressed out he would administer a different general anesthetic to calm me.

The cardiologist proceeded. As before I felt nothing as he inserted the probe in my arm and ran it up and into my heart. Upon getting the probe to the previous stent location, he directed my attention to the X-ray monitor. He showed me the original stents, which were visible on the screen. He pointed out that the two stents were fully occluded, and plugged, which was the reason I was experiencing discomfort and tightness in the chest. He said it appeared the stents appeared to have been plugged for several years. He chuckled and again pointed out that considering the normal expected usefulness of stents is about six to seven years, with mine being in for sixteen and a half years I had gotten more than enough miles out of them. He directed my attention to the monitor. He pointed out that the reason I had not experienced more severe chest pain when the stents were becoming plugged was because, with all my walking, my heart had made its bypass. Over the years my heart has compensated. It had rerouted blood flow to my heart tissue around the blockage. The arteries in my heart in that area were enlarged. In some cases, many times normal size and they had been carrying the blood that could no longer go through the artery with the clogged stents. He studied the x-ray and concluded I had gotten to the point where replacing the stents was no longer an option and that I needed to be examined by a cardiovascular surgeon. That physician would review with me the surgical, bypass options. When the surgeon met with me, he said he needed me to do a stress test to be sure I needed a bypass. He said with the blockage in my heart he was not going to have me do a treadmill test, which could bring upon a real heart attack, but rather he would order the less invasive nuclear stress test to determine my heart output. He said the normal expected output from the heart was 50 to 55 percent of the blood volume with each beat.

The nuclear stress test was done. I asked the technician who administered the test, "how did I do?" The technician was somber, and she did not comment. She said my physician would review the results with me. When I met with the cardiovascular surgeon the next day his expression was dire. I could tell from his concerned look that something was wrong. He acknowledged that the stress test revealed that my heart was only pumping out at a rate of about twenty-five to twenty-six percent which was dangerously low and that I needed immediate surgery. He said because of the low (weak) output of my heart he wanted to admit me as soon as possible to the University hospital. He said there, at that major medical facility, if necessary, he would be able to do a heart transplant if it turned out, my heart could not be saved.

WHAT! A HEART TRANSPLANT! It was all I could do to breathe. He said, before he admitted me to the hospital he wanted to do one last test, an echocardiogram (cardiac ultrasound) diagnostic scan of my heart to verify the results of the previous diagnostic test. He wanted to be sure before he put me in the University hospital for major, lifesaving surgery.

Somewhat in shock, my wife drove me to the echocardiogram test facility the next day. Both of us were afraid of what we were about to find out. Were my days numbered? What was going to be my fate if a donor heart could not be found?

The test room was dark. I was lying on my back on the table. My chest was bare. The test administrator asked if I wanted to watch the test on the monitor and I said most definitely "YES". She swung the screen around so I could see what she was doing. She pointed out that with the test she would be checking the 4 chambers of the heart, and the 4 heart valves and the walls of the heart as well as the blood vessels entering and leaving the heart and the pericardium or sac surrounding the heart. As the test progressed, I could see my heart beating (pulsing). It was going ka-boom, ka-boom, ka-boom. She pointed out the four valves: the mitral valve and the aortic valve. She pointed out how they were opening fully and closing completely, just as they should. Likewise, she pointed out the pulmonary and tricuspid valves which were also opening fully and closing strongly. She showed me the four chambers of my heart and the blood vessels entering and leaving my heart along with the pericardium (the sac surrounding my heart). She moved the scanner around and showed me the scar tissue from my previous heart attack, sixteen plus years before. All the while, I watched as my heart, about the size of a small fist, kept pulsating away rhythmically. I was fascinated. This pump in my body was working, all by itself, with no conscious input from me.

I was mesmerized. Using my fist, I made a strong pumping action. I said to the woman, "that looks like a pretty good heartbeat to me."

Smiling, she quickly replied. She said, "Oh yes, you have a strong heart. A very strong heart. The valves are opening and closing fully just as they should, and the chambers are pumping strongly." Nodding, she smiled. "Yes. It appears you have a very strong and healthy heart."

She told me the test results would be sent to the cardiovascular surgeon's office the next day. Minutes later I left and could barely catch my breath. I was so excited. It was all I could do to keep from running as I proceeded to my car. To this day, I swear I was floating four feet off the ground and had to reach down just to open the car door. When I got in, my wife, the nurse, was taken aback. She said, "You look like you have just seen a miracle. What's going on?"

I told her what the woman who had administered the test had said. I told her what my heart looked like, and I demonstrated with my fist the pumping action I watched. We were both uplifted by what I had seen and learned. Maybe I wouldn't need a transplant after all.

The next day I met with my cardiologist and the cardiovascular surgeon. The surgeon pulled up on his monitor the echocardiogram images to review them with me. He acknowledged the nuclear stress test had been flawed and that I had a very strong heart. One; I did not need a heart transplant. Two; a heart bypass was still advised. If the operation were not performed, I would continue having mild heart attacks until one day a severe one might occur and then I would be in real danger and need emergency bypass surgery. Third; he recommended a triple bypass. He pointed out what artery would be diverted and connected to three arteries in my heart. Fourth; he acknowledged that the bypass operation would be routine, and it did not have to be done at the University hospital. Because a possible heart transplant would no longer be required, he said the by-pass could be done at one of the regional hospitals, but because he had already reserved the operating theater for my surgery, he said he may as well continue with the schedule and do the operation there. He gave me the time I was to be at the hospital and what was expected before admission. He had scheduled me for bypass surgery in two days. All is well and good. He assured me the operation was going to be pretty much routine, and I would be out of the hospital in a week.

The day prior to my surgery, I received a call from the hospital. A couple of emergency heart operations had come up and they needed to delay my surgery two days. I said, "fine." The day prior to the rescheduled surgery I received a call from the hospital, and they asked if it would be okay if they rescheduled my surgery again, again delaying the operation two days. I figured if it was an emergency, I would go along with their request. The day before the third scheduled date, the hospital called again and wanted to reschedule my surgery. I said, "No way. They had rescheduled me twice already and that was enough. I told them I would be arriving at the surgery admitting desk at seven o'clock the next morning and they could do with me as they saw fit, but I was not leaving the hospital until the triple-by-pass operation had been completed.

7:00 AM the next morning I checked in at surgery admitting. Dressed in the surgical gown, I got on the gurney and was wheeled toward the operating suite. The nurse or technician pushing me produced what appeared to be a large oxygen mask that covered my nose and mouth. She said they needed to increase the oxygen level in my blood before surgery, so I needed to take some deep breaths. I took one breath and that was the last thing I remember, until eight hours later when I woke up in a recovery room. My cardiovascular surgeon was standing beside my bed. He was smiling and asked me how I felt. To which I answered, "Okay." I told him I was more than a bit fuzzy, but aside from that I was not in pain."

The surgeon explained that the anesthetic had not yet worn off and I would not feel any pain or discomfort until it did. He said at which time an IV drip would take care of most, if not all, of the ensuing pain. He went on to explain that the two tubes poked into my abdomen were drains and would be removed in a couple days. He described the monitors and IVs connected to me and their function. He said the operation had been a success. He said it had been very straight forward and aside from the fact they had to use fourteen stainless steel wire ties to close the split of my sternum, instead of the customary four wires, because of an osteoporosis issue, the operation had proceeded without a hitch. He said I would be in the intensive care recovery area for a day and then when they were sure I was stable, I would be moved to the coronary care recovery area.

By day four I was up and walking with assistance out into the hall. I would walk the couple dozen feet to the nurses' station and back. By day six, and approaching discharge, I had to prove that I could walk alone the length of the hall without assistance, albeit I was allowed to hold onto my IV and monitor stand. The physical therapist was with me in case I needed assistance, and to keep me from falling, but aside from him being there, I was on my own. Upon getting the green light from my cardiovascular surgeon, and the physical therapy department, that I could be discharged, I was wheeled to the exit. My wife had brought my van around, with chair-height seats that would be easy to get in and out of, and we headed home. At my house, I made the three steps up to the main floor with assistance from my wife. We took it slow, but I made it. Once in the house, I had about enough strength to walk to a bedroom, and that was it. A big sigh of relief; I was home. I had made it through the operation. I was alive and I was home. I was exhausted, but that was expected. I could get in and out of bed, and make it to the bathroom on my own, which was the extent of what I could do that first day home. The next morning, with much help from my wife, I made it up to the kitchen and dining area, one floor above. Using both handrails for support, I made it up the fourteen stairs, without pulling myself along. My surgeon had told me not to lift anything with my arms or pull myself alone with my hands for at least a few weeks. The breastbone needed time to start healing, and the more time it got the better. To be safe, my wife was behind me on the stairs in case I needed support. Initially it t took me nearly ten minutes to make it up the fourteen steps, but I got there. Oh, I was tired, but my surgeon told me that was to be expected. As required, my wife drove me to my first postsurgical doctor visit roughly a week after being discharged. It was a bit of a struggle, getting in and out of the van, but not as bad as I expected. My surgeon checked everything over and said I was progressing on schedule. He told me because they had to use so many wires to tie my breastbone back together, he did not want me touching the steering wheel of my van. It turned out; that he didn't let me drive for four months. He was concerned that the twisting action of my shoulders and arms turning the steering wheel would stress the division of my breastbone and it was better to error on the safe side. With that in mind, I did not drive for over four months and when I started driving again, I limited my adventures to the grocery store and back for over two more months. By then my energy and stamina level had returned. I walked daily, mind you not the six miles I used to do, but a good half to one mile a day.

Post-operation discomfort. Aside from the first five weeks when I could still feel the trauma from having 12 inches of my breastbone split open and pulled apart to expose my heart, and holes poked into my abdomen for the drains, I was on the mend. While I was experiencing some residual pain it was not sufficient for me to renew my pain medication prescription. In fact, the pain I felt was little more than mild discomfort. As a result, I told the cardiovascular surgeon to cancel my prescription for pain pills. I was now on my own, and my strength was slowly coming back. Mind you, not quite to the level of energy and endurance I had a year before the operation, but greater than it had been just before my bypass surgery.

Not until six months had passed since the operation did, I feel I had recovered. I was free of any discomfort and pain of any kind in my chest. I had no angina pain. I was breathing normally. My blood pressure was right where it should be, in the middle of the acceptable range. I was getting around on my own and not exhibiting any outward indications I had a triple bypass operation. I felt good. So, by any standard, the bypass operation was a success.

In summation

As I said upfront, if I knew then what I found out following my first heart attack I would not have had the original heart attack; and quite possibly the follow-on bypass surgery. An old sage once said, 'Too soon old and too late smart'. How true that is. Through this experience, I learned that life is an adventure and not to let a second of it go to waste.

We only have one shot at life, so we need to make the most of every second.

That I plan to do.

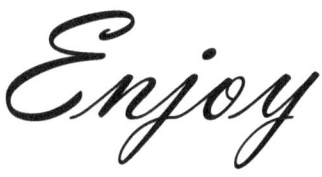

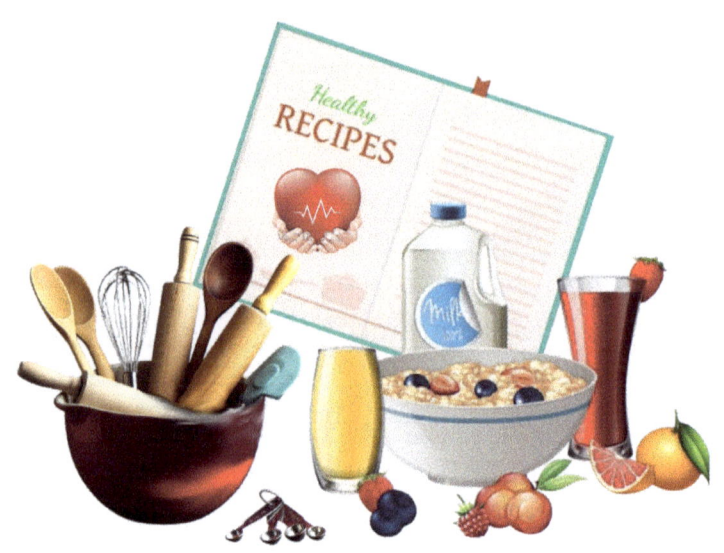

Chapter 12

Receipts

Guide to Eating Properly

The Basics

There are certain fundamentals to managing how much and what we eat. To begin with, there are certain basics needed in the kitchen. The first of which is a good set of measuring cups, the ones that go from a quarter of a cup to one cup. Another is a one-cup and two cup glass measuring cup. The kind you can fill with water and bring to a boil in a microwave. Next is a set of measuring spoons. A lot of readers are going to say, it is only common sense to have a set of each, but you might be surprised how uncommon common sense is. The next is a kitchen scale, one that measures both in ounces and grams. I use the gram setting most as the Nutrition information printed on most packaged products is in grams. All of the recipes below require the use of measuring cups and spoons. And no, a 'dash' of this and two 'dashes' of that or a 'pinch' of this and two 'pinches' of that. That method of measurement is not acceptable.

Recipes

What follows are the recipes I came upon following my initial heart attack. I have since upgraded and polished them, but these are recipes for breakfast, lunches, appetizers, salads, main courses, and desserts that are kind to your heart. I especially focused on recipes that were low in total fat, sodium and sugar, as well as being good for you and a breeze to prepare.

Breakfasts – A great start for the day

Some nutritionists say the most important meal of the day. A good breakfast gets the body and minds off to a hearty start. It wakes everything up. Many of the breakfast items below are simple but important all the same.

Oatmeal. A good place to start and an age-old favorite.

30 Grams/one cup of prepared oatmeal contains 120 Calories, 2 grams of fat, 0 cholesterol, and 4 grams of protein. Add to that 1/3 of a cup of fat-free milk, 30 calories, 0 fat, 5mg cholesterol, 9mg protein, and 13mg of carbohydrate. Top off the oatmeal with 1/2 teaspoon brown sugar substitute (10 calories). Drink the remaining 2/3 of a cup

(130 grams) of the fat free milk and you a have a meal with a total: 220 calories, 2 grams of fat, (from the oatmeal) 5 mg cholesterol from the milk and 13 mg of protein.

Cream of Wheat. In the above recipe substitute cream of wheat for the same amount of oatmeal and most of the above values stay the same. The total calories drop by 10 to 210, and the protein drops from 4 to 3. Aside from that, everything else is the same.

Frozen Breakfast Sandwiches: We have all seen them in the freezer section in the store. But how good are they for us. A close examination of the nutritional facts on the side of the packages is enlightening. Breakfast sandwiches average between 190 to 220 calories per sandwich. Not bad. Most contain somewhere around 8 – 10 grams of total fat. Cholesterol runs around 105mg. Protein is around 9grams and sodium 560 to 600 mg. With a preparation time of about a minute, the frozen sandwiches are a convenient morning breakfast. Add to that a cup (200 grams) of fat free milk, at 90 calories and you have a breakfast with a total of roughly 300 calories, 10 grams of fat, 110 mg cholesterol, 18g protein, and 13g carbohydrate. Time of preparation about 2 minutes.

Dry Cereals. These run the full alphabet gambit from dry flakes to the little 'O' shaped variety. Total calorie wise they vary around 120 to 140 calories per 30gram (one cup serving). Add to that 1 cup of fat free milk (90 grams) and the total calories are 210 to 230, with about 1.5 grams of fat, 5mg of cholesterol, 11g protein and 13g carbohydrate. That is without adding any sugar or sugar substitute. Note: there are some dry breakfast cereals with nuts where the total calories are elevated for the cereal serving alone to upwards of 200 to 250 calories with as much as an additional 3 to 5 grams of fat.

Waffles. The totals of calories for waffles, like with pancakes, varies with the size of the waffle or pancake. For the 7" waffle griddle the calories are between 150 to 180. Add a quarter cup of syrup and the total calories goes up to 400 to 450, plus another 90 calories for a glass (cup/90grams fat free milk) and total calories are at or over 500. Preparation time is obviously greater than pouring a bowl of cereal, but a small price to pay for a hot meal. Add sausages or bacon and the calories will jump even more. This is not a meal I make every morning, and I can afford to occasionally splurge. Preparation time; 15 minutes.

Bran muffins: For those who are bakers I found a nice recipe for bran muffins in the South Beach Diet Cookbook by Arthur Agatston, MD. As stated in their cookbook, 'These satisfying muffins are filled with pieces of pear and spiced with cinnamon.' According to them these muffins freeze well and can be heated individually in a microwave; I suspect in 25 seconds or so. According to them the prep time is about 15 minutes, and the recipe makes a dozen good sized muffins. Nutrition information per individual muffin serving is very good.

Calories per muffin - 130, total fat 5grams, 1/2gram saturated fat, 5 grams protein, 20 grams carbohydrates, 5 grams dietary fiber and 200 mg sodium.

Ingredients:
1-1/2 cups whole-grain pastry flour
1 cup wheat bran
2 tablespoons granular sugar substitute
1-1/4 teaspoon ground cinnamon
1-1/2 teaspoon baking soda
1/4 teaspoon salt
1-1/4 cups 1 percent or fat-free buttermilk
2 large eggs, lightly beaten

3 tablespoons canola oil

1 Bosc pear, cored and cut into ¼" dice

1-1/2 teaspoons vanilla extract

Heat oven to 350 ° F. Line a muffin tin with paper liners or lightly coat with cooking spray. Combine flour, bran, sugar substitute, cinnamon, baking soda, and salt in a large mixing bowl. Combine buttermilk, eggs, oil, pear and vanilla in another mixing bowl. Make a well in the center of the dry ingredients. Add wet ingredients to dry ingredients and mix just to combine, do not over mix. Divide batter evenly into muffin cups. Bake for 20 minutes. Cool and serve. Makes 12.

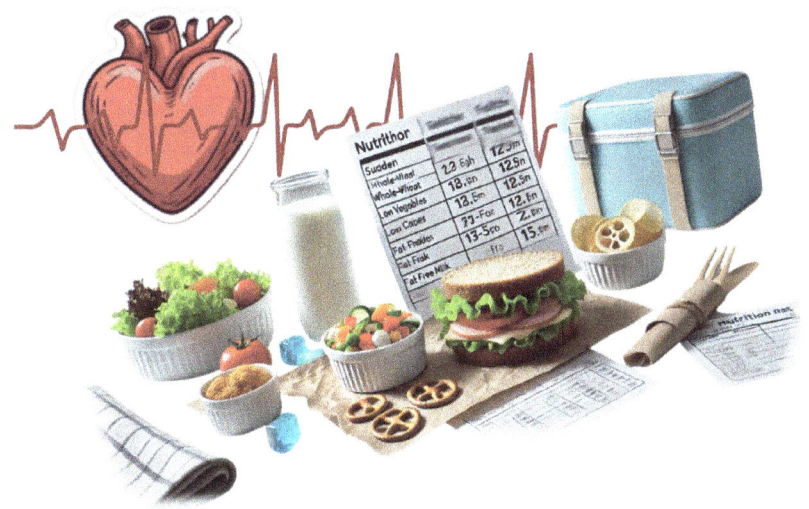

Chapter 13

Lunches

The mid-day meal

So important for those who want to
keep their weight down

One of the things I found out in my studies, the key to good nutrition is three meals a day. Some dietary guides suggest even more small meals a day, but for the busy, work-a-day active person, going from their coffee and a roll for breakfast, a quick grab of anything greasy for lunch and the hitting it BIG at the evening meal or dinner and then snacking until bed time, to three balanced meals is a big improvement. The importance of correct eating three times a day cannot be over stressed. Lunch does not have to be a greasy hamburger and even greasier fries, picked up on the run. Nor need it be a multi-course extravaganza.

Any of the soups and salads listed in the previous sections make marvelous additions to a healthy lunch. The soups can be eaten chilled, or if you have a microwave at work, heated in a minute of two. The salads need to be kept chilled. If you don't have a refrigerator at work, then one of those small coolers will do fine. Put in one of those small refreeze able blue ice packs, a refrigerator-chilled low-fat/low calorie canned drink. Between the two, the salad will stay cool until lunchtime.

If you are going to take a sandwich, make it low-fat whole-wheat bread, lean sliced chicken or turkey or beef with mustard, and light on the low-fat mayonnaise or margarine. The mayonnaise and margarine spread just add calories and a little more to the sandwich in the way of nutrition. For chips there are '*baked*' potato chips with virtually no fat. For desserts, there are any number of fat-free cookies and low-fat, low-calorie puddings. I tried them all and was surprised at how good they tasted and how good I felt when I didn't see the numbers increase when I weighed myself each morning. I was eating healthily and not gaining weight and feeling better than I had in years, not having to pack that extra fifty pounds around.

For lunches, I am beginning with some of the staples listing the calories, fat, cholesterol, carbohydrates, and protein. I have eaten these for years and was never really aware of how many calories, grams of fat, cholesterol, carbohydrates and protein I was eating.

Begin with one everyone knows, the **PB & J**, the venerable **Peanut Butter and Jelly** sandwich. A staple we have all eaten and relayed upon for years. A cinch to prepare - and easy to pack off to work or school.

Contents:

P B & J Sandwich:

2 slices low-fat whole-wheat sandwich bread   100 calories
Fat 2g, 0 cholesterol, 18g carbohydrates, 6g protein

1 tablespoon low-fat or reduced-fat peanut butter   90 calories
Fat 12g, 0 cholesterol, 22 g carbohydrates, 5g protein

1 tablespoon jelly or jam   50 calories
Fat 0, 0 cholesterol, 13g carbohydrates, 0g protein

Chips or crackers:

10 Low sodium potato chips   100 calories
Fat 9g, 0 cholesterol, 16g carbohydrate, 5g protein

2 Reduced-fat Oreo's   100 calories
Fat 4.5g, 0 cholesterol, 27g carbohydrates, 1g protein

1 glass (1 cup) fat free milk   90 calories
Fat 0, 5mg cholesterol, 13g carbohydrates, 9g protein

Totals
Total Calories: 530 calories
Fat 25.5g, 5mg cholesterol, 109g carbohydrates,
26g protein

As a contrast the Lunch meat Sandwich:

Less calories and less fat. A good substitute for the old reliable, P B & J.

There is large range of choices of packaged sliced meats to choose from. For the most part 5 or 6 slices of any of the meats has about the same calories.

1 "Sandwich thin", low-fat whole-wheat roll, equals 2 slices 100 calories
Fat 1g, 0 cholesterol, 22g carbohydrates, 5g protein

5 to 6 slices thin sliced sandwich meat   60 calories
Fat 1g, 25mg cholesterol, 3g carbohydrates, 10g protein

1/4 to 1/2 teaspoon mustard, yellow or spicy   10 calories
Fat 0g, 0 cholesterol, 0g carbohydrates, 0g protein

Snack crackers in lieu of chips:

10 Pretzel thin crisps   100 calories
Fat 1.5g, 0 cholesterol, 22g carbohydrates,
1g dietary fiber, 2g protein

2 Oreo's Reduced-fat   100 calories
Fat 4.5g, 0 cholesterol, 27g carbohydrates,
0g dietary fiber, 1g protein

1 glass (1 cup) fat free milk   90 calories
Fat 0, 5mg cholesterol, 13g carbohydrates, 9g protein

Total Calories: 460 calories
Fat 8g, 30mg cholesterol, 87g carbohydrates, 27g protein

Delicious Tuna Fish Sandwich Filling Sandwich Lunch

A sandwich filling that can be made in minutes and is more than enough for a whole week. Not only good tasting, but also good for you.

1 – 7 oz. can Water Packed Solid White Meat Albacore Tuna. Drain water from the can and then crumble tuna meat into small bits into a medium bowl. Add 1/2 cup dill relish and 2 tablespoons of low-fat mayonnaise. Mix thoroughly.

Makes: 1-3/4 cups sandwich filling, enough for 12 to 13 sandwiches

1 "Sandwich thin", low-fat whole-wheat roll, equals 2 slices 100 calories
Fat 1g, 0 cholesterol, 22g carbohydrates,
5g protein

2 Tablespoons Tuna sandwich filling, evenly spread   22 calories
Fat 1.2g, 12mg cholesterol, 0.3g carbohydrates,
8g protein

Snack crackers in lieu of chips:

10 Pretzel thin crisps   100 calories
Fat 1.5g, 0 cholesterol, 22g carbohydrates,
1g dietary fiber, 2g protein

2 Oreo's Reduced-fat   100 calories
Fat 4.5g, 0 cholesterol, 27g carbohydrates,
0g dietary fiber, 1g protein

1 glass (1 cup) fat free milk   90 calories
Fat 0, 5mg cholesterol, 13g carbohydrates,
9g protein

Total Calories: 412 calories
Fat 8.2g, 17mg cholesterol, 84.3g carbohydrates,
25g protein

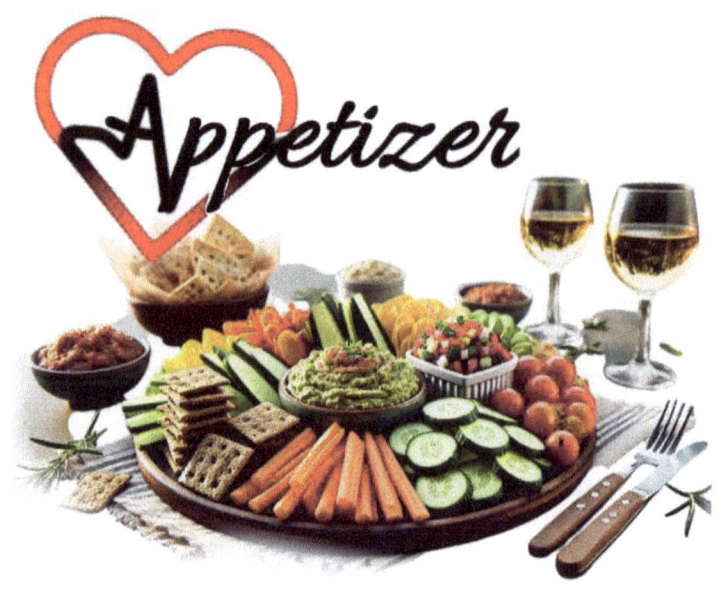

Chapter 14

Appetizers

A delicious introduction to healthy dining

One of the secrets to making a switch to heart healthy eating is the attractive presentation of dishes low in fat and cholesterol. There is no better way to start a casual patio barbecue or a warm congenial sit-down meal than with a delicious appetizer/dip. Always a prelude to good eating when friend's get-together. The appetizer recipes selected are tasty, and easy to prepare.

Delicious Onion Dip

Fantastic with vegetables, low fat baked chips and dippers. A breeze to prepare, and even more fun to eat. Don't be surprised if the bowl is wiped clean.

1 cup fat-free yogurt   1 teaspoon dried dill
1 tablespoon grated onion   1 tablespoon capers
1 tablespoon chopped parsley

Combine all ingredients in a small bowl. Mix thoroughly and chill. Can't be much simpler than that.

Makes one cup

Nutrition Facts   1/4 cup serving contains

Calories:	36	Sodium	126.7 mg
Total Fat:	0.1 g	Carbohydrate	5.1 g
Saturated Fat:	0.1 g	Dietary Fiber	0.1 g
Cholesterol:	1.1 mg	Protein	3.6 g

Chile Pepper Dip

An exciting dip for vegetables, low fat baked chips and dippers. Easy to prepare, and a definite crowd pleaser. A mouth-watering special.

2/3 cup Fat-Free Cottage Cheese

4 tablespoons non-Fat Milk

2 tablespoons Worcestershire

3 teaspoons packaged onion soup mix

1 teaspoon paprika

1 tablespoon onion flakes

14 oz can chopped mild
green Chile peppers

Combine all ingredients a blender or food processor until smooth.

Refrigerate in sealed containers. Makes about one cup

Nutrition Facts		1/4 cup serving contains	
Calories:	57	Sodium	706.2 mg
Total Fat:	0.3 g	Carbohydrate	7.7 g
Saturated Fat:	0.1 g	Dietary Fiber	0.8 g
Cholesterol:	3.7 mg	Protein	6.2 g

Mushroom Crab Delights

Served hot by themselves – combines the woodsy taste of the outdoors with the tangy excitement of crab meat. Serve on crackers or chips. An always crowd pleaser.

24 large mushrooms
1 6oz. can crab meat
1/2 teaspoon paprika
1 celery stalk, finely chopped
1 teaspoon horseradish

1 teaspoons fat-free cream cheese
3 tablespoons pimiento or chopped
   red bell pepper
2 green onions,

Combine shredded crab meat with the cream cheese, chopped pimiento or bell pepper, chopped celery and chopped green onion in a small bowl. Add horseradish and black pepper to suit. Rinse mushrooms, remove stems, and dry on paper towel. Fill mushroom caps with mixture. Dust with paprika. Place on baking sheet and bake at 340F (175C) oven 10 to 12 minutes.

Makes 24
Nutrition Facts   Serving of 3 contains

Calories:	42.6	Sodium	124.5 mg
Total Fat:	0.7 g	Carbohydrate	3.6 g
Saturated Fat:	0.2 g	Dietary Fiber	0.9 g
Cholesterol:	16.5 mg	Protein	6.2 g

Stuffed Tomatoes

Combine the juiciness of fresh red tomatoes with chopped cooked shrimp and you'll have a treat that will have them coming back for more. Best with small tomatoes.

24 small tomatoes	1/4 teaspoons dried mustard
1 6oz. can cocktail shrimp	1/4 cup petite peas - cooked
1/4 cup rice, wild or white	2 tablespoons lemon juice

Season to taste

After slicing the tops off the tomatoes use a small spoon to scoop out the pulp, making tomato shells. Mash tomato pulp and set aside. Halve or quarter shrimp and combine with tomato pulp, rice, mustard, peas and lemon juice. Mix thoroughly. Fill tomato shells with mixture. Cover and refrigerate before serving.

Makes 24

Nutrition Facts		Serving of 3 contains	
Calories:	46.8	Sodium	86.2 mg
Total Fat:	0.5 g	Carbohydrate	5.4 g
Saturated Fat:	0.1 g	Dietary Fiber	1.0 g
Cholesterol:	41.5 mg	Protein	5.4 g

Tempting Pepperoni Cheese Bread

Tempting mini bread pizza treats as delicious as the look. Will disappear with the warm smiles of satisfaction.

1 loaf unsliced French bread
3 ounces Veggie Pepperoni or
   Turkey pepperoni pizza slices

3 tablespoons low-fat
   margarine or vegetable
   spread

6 oz. low-fat mozzarella shredded, or low-fat Monterey jack shredded
3 tablespoons minced parsley for garnish

Slice French bread loaf every 1 inch, leaving the slices attached at the bottom. Brush the melted margarine or softened vegetable spread on both faces of each slice. Place the pepperoni pieces between the slices, sprinkle with the shredded cheese and parsley. Place on ungreased cookie sheet and bake at 350F until cheese is melted, about 12 to 15 minutes.

Makes 24

Nutrition Facts		1 Slice serving contains	
Calories:	91.0	Sodium	229.0 mg
Total Fat:	4.0 g	Carbohydrate	10.0 g
Saturated Fat:	2.0 g	Dietary Fiber	1.0 g
Cholesterol:	12.0 mg	Protein	5.0 g

Zucchini Snacks

A delight exciting way to prepare a popular, but somewhat overlooked member of the squash family, that can be both delectable and good for you.

Half dozen medium sized zucchini	1 teaspoons basil
4 oz. pack crumbled blue cheese	1/3 cup parmesan cheese
10 to 12 cherry tomatoes – sliced in thin slices	

Slice zucchini into 1/2" to 3/4" sections. Scoop out half of the insides leaving the bottom in place. Discard the scooped-out zucchini pulp. Place the zucchini on an ungreased cookie sheet. Fill the hollowed-out center in the zucchini with the crumbled blue cheese, level to the top. Place a tomato slice on top and sprinkle with the parmesan cheese and basil. Add black pepper to taste.
Bake at 400F until cheese is melted, about 5 to 7 minutes.
Serve straight from the oven.

Makes about 3 dozen.

For an interesting change of pace, substitute shredded jalapeño pepper cheese. Also, slice the zucchini into 1/2" thick slices, hollow out the center completely, place on tomato slice and fill level, place another tomato slice and fill level, place another thin slice of tomato on top, sprinkle the parmesan and bake.

Nutrition Facts		Serving of 2 snacks contains	
Calories:	38.0	Sodium	116.0 mg
Total Fat:	2.0 g	Carbohydrate	2.0 g
Saturated Fat:	2.0 g	Dietary Fiber	trace
Cholesterol:	6.0 mg	Protein	2.0 g

Lemon Skinny Dip

Excellent with vegetables, low fat baked chips and dippers. An exciting dip that can also work well as a salad dressing.

2 cups fat-free sour cream   1/4 cup non fat milk
1 pack vanilla pudding mix   4 teaspoon lemon juice
1 teaspoon lemon peel grated

Combine all ingredients in a bowl and whisk until blended. Chill.

Makes 2 cups

For a less tart dip, add 1 to 2 tablespoons sugar.

Nutrition Facts   1/4 cup serving contains

Calories:	95.6	Sodium	191.4 mg
Total Fat:	5.3 g	Carbohydrate	7.5 g
Saturated Fat:	3.8 g	Dietary Fiber	trace
Cholesterol:	20.2 mg	Protein	4.5 g

Salsa Excitement

Especially good with vegetables, low fat baked chips and dippers.

1 cup chopped fresh tomatoes	1/2	teaspoon oregano
1/3 cup chopped jalapeno chilies	1	tablespoon chopped cilantro
3 medium white onion chopped	1	tablespoon fresh lime juice

Combine all ingredients in a small bowl. Season to taste with black pepper. Refrigerate in a cover container.

Makes about 1-1/2 cups.

Nutrition Facts		1/4 cup serving contains	
Calories:	35.0	Sodium	102.0 mg
Total Fat:	1.0 g	Carbohydrate	6.5 g
Saturated Fat:	0.2 g	Dietary Fiber	1.0 g
Cholesterol:	0.2 mg	Protein	1.0 g

Two Bean Dip

Out of this world with low fat baked chips and dippers
1/2 cup fat-free yogurt
1/2 cup "Fantastic Salsa Excitement"
1/2 teaspoons garlic powder, (not garlic salt)
1/2 teaspoon chili powder
1 cup cooked & drained kidney and pinto beans

Combine yogurt, salsa, garlic powder, and chili powder in a small bowl and stir until blended. Coarse chop beans. Stir beans into blended mixture. Refrigerate in sealed container.
Makes 2 cups

Nutrition Facts		1/4 cup serving contains	
Calories:	48.0	Sodium	39.0 mg
Total Fat:	0.4 g	Carbohydrate	8.6 g
Saturated Fat:	0.1 g	Dietary Fiber	1.8 g
Cholesterol:	0.3 mg	Protein	3.1 g

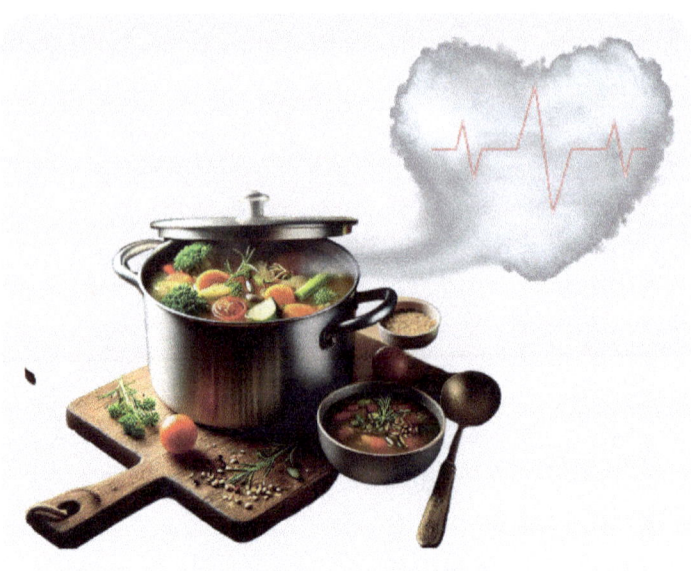

Chapter 15

Soups

A traditional beginning to a balanced meal

Simple to prepare. Convenient to serve. An ideal microwaveable – reheat able quick pick-me-up kind of addition to a meal - or the makings of a well-rounded lunch. And like with the appetizers, the recipes selected are tasty, low in fat, quick to prepare and good for you. You'll find these soups are great steamy on a cold, blustery day. They are guaranteed to warm you through and through. But don't stop when the thermometer outside starts to climb as many of the following recipes are great chilled on a sultry hot day as well. Try them. You will like them, especially because they won't add inches to the waistline.

Unlike many recipe collections, I have tried to focus on those which do not require advanced culinary skills. To prepare most of the recipes included here will require little more than the most basic cooking ability.

Another point I need to make regards salt. People with diagnosed coronary artery disease need to subscribe to the axiom, *"Salt is an acquired taste. Stop adding salt to foods for a month and be surprised how you can shake the habit."* As a result, you will notice salt was not included in any of the recipes. How can that be done? Simple, the ingredients alone in most dishes contain all the salt needed without the addition of extra. Make the recipe and taste it before adding salt. Try it without and then if salt is required, keep it to a minimum.

Colorful Carrot Soup

A different soup that will get smiles of approval. A taste sensation with a tangy hint of onion. Another soup that serves well as a microwaveable lunch meal.

1-1/2 cups shredded carrots	1 tablespoon rice
1/2 cup chopped onion	1 tablespoon margarine
1 quart fat-free broth	1 cup frozen baby peas
1/4 cup tomato sauce or paste	

Combine carrots, onion, broth, rice, margarine, and tomato sauce in large, 4-quart sauce pan. Stirring constantly, bring to a boil. Turn heat down to simmer and cover. Stir occasionally and simmer for 30 to 40 minutes. Add the frozen baby peas.

Makes 6 Servings

Garnish with bacon bits, a sprig of parsley or pinch of chopped chives and a twist of course ground pepper.

Nutrition Facts   1 cup serving contains

Calories:	60.0	Sodium	160.0 mg
Total Fat:	0.4 g	Carbohydrate	12.5 g
Saturated Fat:	0.1 g	Dietary Fiber	2.5 g
Cholesterol:	0.0 mg	Protein	2.6 g

Traditional Split-Pea Soup

Great any time of the year as a take to work microwaveable lunch entry. Few will disagree there is nothing like a bowl of thick pea soup to warm the soul on a cool evening before a relaxing meal. With less than one gram of fat and a fraction of a gram of saturated fat, what could be healthier? And remember, try it without salt first – you will be surprised.

2 cups dried split peas	4 carrots quartered & sliced
3 cups water	4 celery stalks quartered & sliced
6 bouillon cubes	2 bay leaves
1 garlic clove, chopped	1/2 teaspoon thyme
1 onion sliced and chopped	2 tablespoons bacon bits
Course ground pepper to suit	Salt if absolutely needed

Place peas in colander and rinse with cold water. Place rinsed peas in large pot, 4 quart recommended. Pour in the water and add bouillon cubes, a garlic, onion, carrots, celery, bay leaves, thyme and real bacon bits. Bring to boil, stirring frequently. Reduce heat to simmer and cover. Simmer until vegetables are tender, about 45 to 55 minutes.

Makes about 8 Servings

Garnish each bowl with a twist of coarse ground pepper, followed by a 1/4 teaspoon real bacon bits, topped with a bay leaf for color.

Nutrition Facts		1 cup serving contains	
Calories:	202.0	Sodium	902.0 mg
Total Fat:	0.9 g	Carbohydrate	36.5 g
Saturated Fat:	0.2 g	Dietary Fiber	5.6 g
Cholesterol:	0.5 mg	Protein	13.4 g

Traditional Navy-Bean Soup

Not something you will find in many stores, but a soup well worth the minimal effort to prepare. A soup that some say is better reheated, so make enough to reheat tomorrow.

2 cups Navy beans - dry
2 quarts water
1 small onion chopped

1 garlic clove
1 bay leaf

Wash Navy beans with cold water in colander. Place beans in large pot, 4 quarts or larger, and add water, covering beans 3 to 4 inches. Bring to a boil for 2 minutes. Remove from heat and cover and let cool for 2 hours. Drain beans and discard soaking water. Add 2 quarts of water, chopped onion garlic, clove and bay leaf and bring to boil. Cover and simmer until beans are tender, about 2 hours.

Makes 8 Servings

Season to suit with course ground pepper.

<u>Nutrition Facts</u>   <u>1 cup serving contains</u>

Calories:	75.0	Sodium	40.0 mg
Total Fat:	0.3 g	Carbohydrate	14.0 g
Saturated Fat:	0.1 g	Dietary Fiber	4.5 g
Cholesterol:	0.0 mg	Protein	4.5 g

Fantastic Chili

So good and so tasty - few will take the time to notice there's no beef. Filled with beans, tomatoes, ground turkey, and a ton of flavor; even die-hard beef chili lovers will come back for more. A great warm and filling addition to any winter meal. Still, it is especially good as the summer cook-out or barbecue. A healthy selection that will draw smiles any time of the year.

1-1/2 lb lean ground turkey.	1- 6 oz can tomato sauce
2 onions chopped	1 tablespoon chili powder
1-1/2 teaspoons oregano	1 tablespoon baking cocoa
1-1/2 teaspoons cumin	1/2 teaspoon salt
1 28oz can diced tomatoes	1/4 teaspoon cinnamon
3 15oz cans kidney beans	3 cups low fat beef broth
Rinsed and drained	3 - 4 bay leaves

In a large pot cook the turkey and onions over medium heat until the meat is no longer pink. Drain and discard the liquid. Mix in the oregano and cumin. Add the diced tomatoes, broth, tomato sauce, chili powder, cocoa, salt, cinnamon and bay leaves. Stir and bring to a boil. Reduce heat and cover. Simmer for 30 to 45 minutes. Add beans and continue to simmer for another 30 to 45 minutes.

Makes about 12 – 1 cup Servings

Nutrition Facts		1 cup serving contains	
Calories:	276.0	Sodium	900.0 mg
Total Fat:	6.0 g	Carbohydrate	34.5 g
Saturated Fat:	1.0 g	Dietary Fiber	13.0 g
Cholesterol:	45.0 mg	Protein	22.0 g

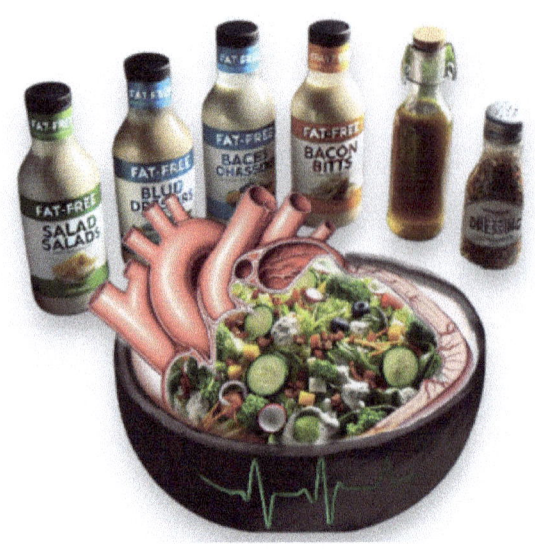

Chapter 16

Salads

Filled with vitamins - High in Fiber

Always a tasty addition to a healthy meal

S alads know no limit. If you haven't looked lately, the selection of 'Fat-free' salad dressings is in the store is tremendous. It covers the full spectrum from blue cheese to ranch. All the traditional are there. Admittedly some brands are taster than others, but that is a matter of personal taste. With many brands it's difficult to tell them from the old stand-by fat filled varieties.

I had fun trying all the '*Fat-free*' salad dressings and picking the ones I liked the best. I experimented with different types of lettuce and greens. I garnished the salads with vegetables and '*Fat-free*' croutons. I had fun checking out the new designer salad dressings from the small specialty producers. Turns out those small producers have come out with some very exciting new tastes.

Some of the tips I learned when preparing salads.

1. 1Rinse the lettuce or greens in cold water and spin dry. When I didn't have a salad/lettuce spinner available I'd pat the greens dry with paper towels. Wet lettuce will dilute the dressing.

2. 2Following that I would chill the lettuce and greens in the refrigerator before preparing the salad. That I learned to maintain crispness.

3. I would chill the bowls and plates before serving; that too helps the salad crisp.

4. For eye appeal and a spark of added flavor I would garnish with crumbled or shredded cheese, ground whole pepper, bacon bits or diced vegetables for added pizzazz.

Traditional Potato Salad

A staple summer pleaser. What would a picnic or barbeque be without chilled creamy potato salad. We are expected to serve it so why not serve a potato salad that is not only good for us but that tastes good as well. My family and guests could not believe a potato salad with so much flavor could be low in fat and good for us at the same time.

3 cups sliced, cooked and peeled potatoes
1/2 cup chopped dill pickles
1/4 cup chopped green onions
2 teaspoons dried parsley
1 tablespoon dried parsley
1 tablespoon dry mustard

1/3 cup fat-free mayonnaise
1/4 cup fat-free plain yogurt
2 sliced radishes
1/4 cup chopped green bell
    pepper

Combine all ingredients in a large bowl. Stir until thoroughly mixed. Chill 2 hours and serve on chilled plates for best results.

Makes about 5 Servings

Season to suit with course ground pepper.

Nutrition Facts		a serving contains	
Calories:	169.0	Sodium	486.6 mg
Total Fat:	4.4 g	Carbohydrate	30.5 g
Saturated Fat:	0.8 g	Dietary Fiber	2.8 g
Cholesterol:	5.3 mg	Protein	3.7 g

Zany Tuna Salad

Add eye appeal and palate pleasing adventure to a salad that is sure to satisfy even the most difficult in any group, and a chinch to prepare.

8 oz pack of elbow macaroni	1 cup dried celery
9 oz can water packed tuna, chunks drained	1 cup fat-free mayonnaise
1 oz can mandarin oranges drained	1 teaspoon lemon juice
1 cup chopped peeled apple	1/4 teaspoon salt

Cook macaroni per instructions on package. Drain and rinse with cold water and place in large bowl. Add tuna chunks, orange chunks, chopped apple, and diced celery. In a medium bowl mix together the fat-free mayonnaise, lemon juice, and salt. Fold the mayonnaise mixture into the combined ingredients in large bowl. Garnish with paprika and cover and refrigerate 3 to 4 hours.

Nutrition Facts		3/4 cup serving contains	
Calories:	176.0	Sodium	453.0 mg
Total Fat:	1.0 g	Carbohydrate	27.0 g
Saturated Fat:	0.1 g	Dietary Fiber	1.0 g
Cholesterol:	9.0 mg	Protein	13.0 g

Swimming with delight Shrimp Salad

Not your ordinary shrimp salad, but one that is guaranteed to bring your family and guests back for seconds. No cooking required; just mix and stir. Great with tiny cocktail shrimp, but equally as good with crab meat or salmon chunks.

12 oz cocktail shrimp	1 tablespoon lemon juice
1/4 cup chili or cocktail sauce	1 tablespoon dried horseradish
1/2 cup fat-free yogurt	1 celery stalk chopped

Combine chili sauce and yogurt in a large bowl. Add shrimp, lemon juice, horseradish and celery. Chill until ready to serve. Line salad bowl with lettuce leaves and spoon in salad mixture. Garnish with a halved cherry tomato and asparagus spears.

Makes 4 to 5 servings

Nutrition Facts   each serving contains

Calories:	150.0	Sodium	38.0 mg
Total Fat:	2.3 g	Carbohydrate	11.0 g
Saturated Fat:	0.5 g	Dietary Fiber	3.2 g
Cholesterol:	6.0 mg	Protein	23.0 g

Tomato Lovers Salad

Not for everyone, but for those who are into fresh tomatoes and like a salad filled with delightful tastes, this is the salad for them.

2 tomatoes chopped into chunks
1 cucumber seeded and chopped
1 small onion chopped
3 cups cooked rice, chilled

2 tablespoons olive oil
2 tablespoons cider vinegar
2 teaspoon basil
1/4 teaspoon pepper

Combine oil, vinegar, basil and pepper. Mix until uniform. Add tomatoes, cucumbers, onion and rice. Toss until evenly mixed. Chill and serve.

Makes about 6 to 8 servings

Nutrition Facts   each serving contains

Calories:	118.0	Sodium	5.0 mg
Total Fat:	4.1 g	Carbohydrate	19.5 g
Saturated Fat:	1.1 g	Dietary Fiber	1.0 g
Cholesterol:	0.0 mg	Protein	2.0 g

Chilled Bean Salad

A quick and simple salad that is easy to prepare and a nice addition to any picnic table or family get-together. Don't be afraid to double the recipe. You can never make too much of this summertime standard.

1 cup kidney or black beans cooked & drained	2 tablespoons wine vinegar
2 celery stalks chopped	3 small onions chopped
1/2 bell pepper chopped	2 tablespoons olive oil
1/4 cup sliced green olives	1 tablespoon dried parsley
3 tablespoons pimiento chopped	

Combine all ingredient in a large bowl. Mix until thoroughly combined. Chill for 2 hours. Serve chilled. Garnish with pimiento.

Makes about 4 servings

Nutrition Facts   each serving contains

Calories:	137.0	Sodium	113.0 mg
Total Fat:	7.5 g	Carbohydrate	13.5 g
Saturated Fat:	1.1 g	Dietary Fiber	3.5 g
Cholesterol:	0.0 mg	Protein	4.5 g

Super Cool Pasta Salad

Another salad specialty easy to make, and always a crowd favorite. Great for summer cookouts where something cool hits the spot.

2 cups cooked pasta	1 carrot peeled & chopped
1 sliced cucumber	2 celery stalks sliced
1 cup chopped broccoli	3 oz can chicken chunks
1 bell pepper chopped	1/3 cup fat-free Italian dressing

Combine in a large bowl, pasta, cucumber, broccoli, chopped bell pepper, carrot, celery and chicken chunks. Pour Italian dressing over mixture and stir until thoroughly mixed. Chill until ready to serve. Garnish with carrots.

Makes about 6 servings

Nutrition Facts   each serving contains

Calories:	200.0	Sodium	220.0 mg
Total Fat:	9.3 g	Carbohydrate	18.5 g
Saturated Fat:	1.1 g	Dietary Fiber	4.0 g
Cholesterol:	12.0 mg	Protein	10.5 g

Oriental Bean Salad

A light and easy lunch take-along. Best to keep chilled or refrigerated until lunch time. Can be served right out of the refrigerator or microwaved for a minute to warm up. For a little extra pizzazz add a little ground bacon bits.

1 cup white or wild rice	1 small can kidney beans
1-1/2 cups water	1/2 cup orange juice
Pinch of salt	2 tablespoons lemon juice
1 cup chopped peeled mango	1 tablespoon low fat margarine
1/2 finely chopped sweet red pepper	

In a medium saucepan bring the water, orange juice, margarine and salt to a boil. Add the rice and simmer until the rice is tender and most of the liquid is gone, about 15 to 20 minutes maximum. Remove from heat. Pour rice into colander and rinse with cold water. Set rice aside to drain. Drain the kidney beans and pour into a large mixing bowl. Add the mango, chopped sweet red pepper and lime juice and mix together. Add the rice and mix thoroughly. Refrigerate until ready to serve. Served chilled or microwave.

Makes about 6 servings

Add a 1/4 cup of cooked bacon bits for a little extra texture and flavor.

Nutrition Facts		each serving contains	
Calories:	225.0	Sodium	280.0 mg
Total Fat:	3.0 g	Carbohydrate	67.0 g
Saturated Fat:	1.1 g	Dietary Fiber	2.0 g
Cholesterol:	2.0 mg	Protein	3.4 g

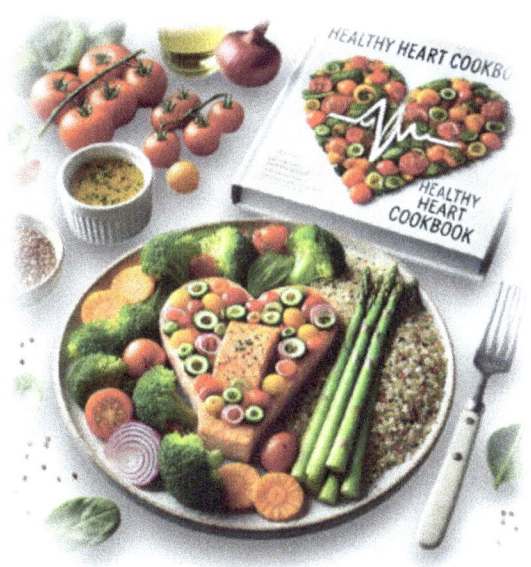

Chapter 17

Dinners

The evening meal

A time to savor the day's events and enjoy a relaxing meal.

The 'low fat', 'low cholesterol' options are endless. I have tried to select recipes based on ease of preparation and taste appeal. My intent has been to make a friendly understanding of what I did toward the goal of better health and a satisfying lifestyle. With twenty plus years since my first heart attack and later triple bypass surgery and still going strong has to be some accomplishment.

While I was aware many people enjoy puttering in the kitchen, I am like many folks who work full-time and don't have the time and energy in the evening to prepare large, extravagant meals. I have listed some tasty recipes that focus on ease of preparation and are a joy to eat.

The first recipe I have selected has been a favorite of ours for years and I feel confident you too will find it tasty and a breeze to prepare. Included in this section are recipes for salsa and barbeque sauce that can be used to enhance the flavor and create a taste sensation of an otherwise ordinary meal. Many of the fish and fowl recipes I have selected can be prepared with a variety of meat selections, thereby providing several options with one recipe.

Cranberry Chicken

One of the simplest evening meals. A main dish that takes a few minutes to prepare. Its taste is exciting and something people don't tire of easily. The great part about this dish is that while it is baking you have the time to prepare some rice and a simple lettuce salad to round out the meal. Add a serving of peas or other vegetables and the dinner is complete.

4 chicken breasts skinned and boned with fat removed.
16 oz can cranberry sauce, whole
2 tablespoons juice of an orange
1 teaspoon grated orange peel
2 tablespoons honey
1/2 teaspoon allspice

Preheat oven to 375 F. In a small bowl stir together cranberry sauce, orange juice, honey, and allspice. Trim all fat from chicken breasts and place in baking dish. Pour 1/2 of the mixture over the chicken. Bake on one side for 15 minutes. Turn the chicken breasts and pour remainder of mixture over chicken. Bake second side for 30 to 35 minutes. Serve with rice and peas. Pour mixture from baking dish over rice.

Makes about 4 servings

Nutrition Facts		each serving contains	
Calories:	225.0	Sodium	70.0 mg
Total Fat:	3.2 g	Carbohydrate	36.5 g
Saturated Fat:	1.0 g	Dietary Fiber	0.7 g
Cholesterol:	72.0 mg	Protein	24.5 g

Super Tropical Mahimahi

A no skill required fish dish that takes but a few minutes to prepare. Astonish your family or guests with a wildly exciting, pallet pleasing meal, that's impressive yet so simple to prepare. Pan seared fish fillets served atop spinach or lettuce leaves sprinkled with a salsa of your choice. This is equally good with other firm fish such as tuna, halibut, shark, tilapia. Try them all for variety. I usually pickup what the local butcher says is the freshest. It turns out, they all taste great.

1 4oz fish fillet per person	1/4 teaspoon salt
Fat free cooking spray	1/4 teaspoon pepper

Preheat a large electric nonstick fry pan to 400F or preheat a nonstick stove top skillet on high until hot. Sprinkle fish with a hint of salt and pepper. Put fish on waxed paper to protect kitchen counter and spray both sides of fish liberally with cooking spray. Remove fish from waxed paper and place on preheated skillet. Sear each side until brown. About 1 minute per side. Reduce heat to medium and cook uncovered until fish flakes easily when tested with a fork, about 7 to 8 minutes. Cooking time will vary slightly depending on thickness of fish fillets.

Nutrition Facts - 4 oz Mahimahi   each serving contains

Calories:	120.0	Sodium	53.0 mg
Total Fat:	1.0 g	Carbohydrate	0.0 g
Saturated Fat:	0.3 g	Dietary Fiber	0.0 g
Cholesterol:	49.0 mg	Protein	32.5 g

Nutrition Facts - 4 oz Tilapia   each serving contains

Calories:	144.0	Sodium	59.0 mg
Total Fat:	3.0 g	Carbohydrate	0.0 g
Saturated Fat:	0.9 g	Dietary Fiber	0.0 g
Cholesterol:	59.0 mg	Protein	39.3 g

For tuna, halibut, shark the nutrition values vary slightly, also ounces of fish matters.
Serve on spinach leaves topped with salsa. Exquisite to look at and even better to eat. Check out salsa on next page that is a breeze to make.

Speedy No Cook Salsa

Great on meat dishes and as a topping on baked potato and as a snack dip.

An easy salsa that goes together in minutes. A breeze to prepare and a sure crowd pleaser. Not too hot with a nice mellow flavor.

1 cup peeled and diced papaya, about a half a medium papaya
3 tablespoons finely chopped red onion
2/3 cup chopped fresh pineapple
2 tablespoons chopped cilantro
1 kiwifruit, peeled and chopped
2 tablespoons pineapple juice
1 jalapeno pepper seeded and minced

Combine all ingredients in a large bowl. Mix thoroughly and cover and refrigerate. Keep chilled until served.

Makes about 4 servings

Nutrition Facts		each 1/2 cup serving contains	
Calories:	15.0	Sodium	1.0 mg
Total Fat:	0.0 g	Carbohydrate	3.8 g
Saturated Fat:	0.0 g	Dietary Fiber	0.6 g
Cholesterol:	0.0 mg	Protein	0.5 g

Magnificent Meatballs

One of those dishes that can be made hours or even a day before. Less than an hour prep time, a main dish that will be the it of any meal at home or away. These are also great for the summer picnic where you want to take something everyone will like and is easy to transport and even easier to reheat and serve. Depending on taste, lean ground pork can be substituted for the lean ground turkey.

3/4 pound lean ground beef	3/4 cup fat free bread crumbs
3/4 pound lean ground turkey	1/4 cup dried onion flakes
2 egg whites	2 tablespoons dried mustard
1/4 cup fat-free milk	1/4 teaspoon salt
1/4 cup red wine	1 cup barbecue sauce

Blend meat together in a large mixing bowl. Mix in eggs, milk, bread crumbs, onion flakes, mustard and salt. Mix well. Roll into 1-1/4" balls. Place meat balls in a nonstick electric fry pan or nonstick stove top fry pan and cook at medium high temperature until meat is no longer pink. Reduce heat to simmer and add 1/4 cup red wine and barbecue sauce and cook for at least 30 minutes.

Serve alone or over yolk free noodles or pasta.

Makes about 36 meatballs

Nutrition Facts   each 6 meatball serving contains

Calories:	560.0	Sodium	120.0 mg
Total Fat:	12.3 g	Carbohydrate	98.5 g
Saturated Fat:	3.7 g	Dietary Fiber	4.0 g
Cholesterol:	62.0 mg	Protein	30.5 g

Great Escape Barbecue Marinade Sauce

Ever get caught without your favorite barbecue marinade, I have. Don't fret. I came upon a recipe that is quick and easy to make and with a blend of tastes that can't be matched. It turns out the spices chosen compliment one another and make for an unbelievable tasty seasoning. This marinade takes but minutes to make and friends and relatives alike will demand the recipe. A secret. This marinade goes real well on beef burgers, but also compliments veggie burgers as well as chicken breasts.

1/3 cup honey	1/4 teaspoon cayenne
1/4 cup low sodium soy sauce	1/4 teaspoon paprika
1/4 cup olive oil	1/4 teaspoon allspice
1 tablespoons vinegar	

Combine all ingredients in a medium bowl and mix thoroughly. Put in medium left-over dish and cover and refrigerate. Keep chilled until used.

Makes about 1 cup

Nutrition Facts		each 1/4 cup serving contains	
Calories:	194.0	Sodium	501.0 mg
Total Fat:	3.5 g	Carbohydrate	19.8 g
Saturated Fat:	0.5 g	Dietary Fiber	0.0 g
Cholesterol:	0.0 mg	Protein	0.3 g

Barbecue Chicken, Turkey, or Burgers

Using the barbecue marinade sauce just described, it is time to experiment. To do this won't even require an outdoor grill. Fantastic creations can be prepared right on the stove, regardless of the weather outside.

4 oz chicken breasts or
4 oz turkey breasts or
Veggie burgers

Place the chicken or turkey breasts or veggie patties in a single layer in a baking dish. Pour about a cup of barbecue marinade sauce in the dish and thoroughly coat both sides of each breast. Cover, refrigerate and let stand for at least an hour. This can actually be done hours in advance, 15 minutes before dinner is planned place the chicken or turkey breasts or veggie burgers on a grill over a medium hot setting, or on an electric fry pan set at 300 degrees. Coat each with more of the marinade and turn frequently until meat is no longer pink when cut.

Nutrition Facts   each chicken breast contains

Calories:	190.0	Sodium	270.0 mg
Total Fat:	5.0 g	Carbohydrate	12.8 g
Saturated Fat:	2.0 g	Dietary Fiber	0.0 g
Cholesterol:	72.6 mg	Protein	28.3 g

Nutrition Facts   each turkey breast contains

Calories:	228.0	Sodium	324.0 mg
Total Fat:	6.0 g	Carbohydrate	14.2 g
Saturated Fat:	2.6 g	Dietary Fiber	0.0 g
Cholesterol:	63.8 mg	Protein	24.7 g

Baked Bean Adventure

If you are like me and occasionally get tired of the old regular baked bean dishes that leave us asking where's the meat, then here is a dish that will take care of that. This baked bean dish is different and will have everyone coming back asking for more. It is simple to prepare. Let your slow cooker do all the work.

2 16 oz cans navy beans	1 large finely chopped onion
1 15 oz can kidney beans	1 medium chopped green bell pepper
2 14 oz cans diced tomatoes	1 garlic clove, minced
1 pound lean ground beef	1/4 cup brown sugar packed
1 cup barbecue sauce	2 tablespoons BBQ sauce, salt free

Cook ground beef in electric fry pan until crumbled and no pink showing. Turn off heat and immediately drain fat and discard. In a large 5-quart slow cooker, combine crumbled cooked beef with remaining ingredients. Stir thoroughly and cook on highest setting for one hour. Reduce heat to low cooking setting and cook for 6 to 8 hours.

Makes about 10 servings

Nutrition Facts		each 1 cup serving contains	
Calories:	215.0	Sodium	645.0 mg
Total Fat:	2.0 g	Carbohydrate	35.8 g
Saturated Fat:	0.9 g	Dietary Fiber	2.6 g
Cholesterol:	22.0 mg	Protein	16.5 g

Sultry Fish Steaks - Salmon, Tuna

A delightful and easy way to prepare any fish steaks. Pick the fish that the butcher nods as being the freshest and do your magic. In minutes you can create a meal that will get you raves and applause. It is so simple to prepare, you will wonder why you hadn't tried it before. And the beauty of this recipe it works well with so many types of fish steaks. Salmon, tuna, halibut.

4 4 oz fish steaks	1/2 cup low fat Monterey Jack Cheese - shredded
1 tablespoons olive or canola oil	1/4 teaspoon sage
1/2 cup mild salsa	1/8 teaspoon pepper
Basil leaves	1/4 teaspoon salt

In a nonstick electric skillet or fry pan heat oil to a medium heat. Cook the fish steaks 3 minutes on each side or until the fish flakes with a fork. Sprinkle the fish with the sage, pepper and salt. Place a couple of basil leaves on each fish steak and spoon on the salsa. Cover with shredded Monterey Jack cheese and cover. Cook on low heat until cheese is melted, about 5 to 8 minutes. Serve with rice, string beans and a slice of pineapple for color.

Serves 4

Nutrition Facts   each fish serving alone contains

Calories:	186.0	Sodium	345.0 mg
Total Fat:	6.0 g	Carbohydrate	2.8 g
Saturated Fat:	1.0 g	Dietary Fiber	0.0 g
Cholesterol:	48.0 mg	Protein	23.0 g

Vintage Veal Cutlet

A taste dish that takes but a few minutes to prepare. Always a family and dinner guest favorite. Just add a helping of wild rice or a boiled potato and the meal is complete.

4 veal cutlets	3 small zucchini sliced
1 8 oz package of sliced mushrooms	2 garlic cloves mince
1/2 cup Monterey Jack cheese grated	1 cup white or red wine
1/2 cup sliced green olives	salt & pepper

Coat the zucchini with cooking spray and place the zucchini and garlic in a nonstick electric fry pan. Cook on medium heat (300F) until tender, about 3 to 4 minutes. Set zucchini aside in a small pan and keep warm. Bring the fry pan up to medium heat again. Coat mushrooms with cooking spray and place in fry pan. Stir constantly and cook until golden brown, about 4 minutes. Then add wine, onions, salt and pepper to taste. Cook until most of liquid is absorbed, about 3 to 4 minutes. Set mushroom mixture aside in another small pan and keep warm. Coat veal with cooking spray and place in skillet now set on high heat. Brown each side for 1minute. Reduce to low heat. Add wine and simmer for 2 minutes or until liquid no longer bubbles. Add mushrooms and zucchini and simmer on low heat until ready to serve.

To serve, spoon mushroom and liquid over cutlets, with zucchini on the side. Add rice or boiled potatoes to round out the meal.

Makes 4 servings

Nutrition Facts		each cutlet alone contains	
Calories:	238.0	Sodium	530.0 mg
Total Fat:	10.0 g	Carbohydrate	6.8 g
Saturated Fat:	4.3 g	Dietary Fiber	1.6 g
Cholesterol:	107.0 mg	Protein	30.5 g

Chicken Orange Delight

Everyone loves chicken, it's the old standby. So why not make it a little different. Zip it up with the delightful flavor of orange. Your guest and family will be impressed, and it will be as good and tasty as it is good for you and the waistline. A cinch to prepare. Baking in the oven does most of the work.

4 chicken breasts boned & skinned	2 tablespoons sauce
1/2 cup corn flakes crumbled	1-1/2 teaspoons paprika
1/3 cup orange juice concentrate	1 teaspoon water
1/2 teaspoon grated orange peel	2 teaspoons basil
1 package imitation butter granules	1/4 cup egg substitute

Clean all visible fat from chicken breasts. Combine corn flakes, paprika, orange peel and basil on a large dinner plate. In a pie plate stir together egg substitute, low sodium soy sauce, water, butter granules and thawed orange concentrate. Mix thoroughly. Preheat oven to 375F. Spray baking sheet with non-fat butter-flavored cooking spray. Dip chicken breasts in egg/orange concentrate, mixture and then roll the chicken in the crumbs. Place coated chicken on baking sheet. Bake until done all the way through, about 30 to 40 minutes.

Makes 4 servings

Nutrition Facts		each 4 oz chicken breast contains	
Calories:	214.0	Sodium	755.0 mg
Total Fat:	2.0 g	Carbohydrate	15.8 g
Saturated Fat:	1.0 g	Dietary Fiber	0.4 g
Cholesterol:	72.2 mg	Protein	36.3 g

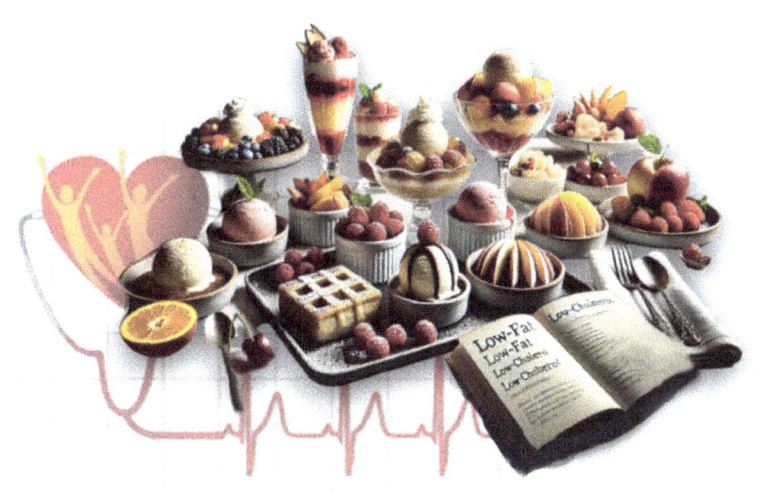

Chapter 18

Desserts

The treat we have all been waiting for.

What better way to end a healthy meal than to treat yourself to a delicious dessert that's exciting to look at as well as delicious and healthy for you.

Desserts are supposed to be a joy. They should be as much fun to eat as they are to prepare. In this section I have tried to select recipes that are easy to fix and are as much as a feast to the eye as they are to the pallet. As I have said before, my recipe selection is geared toward the working person who wants to eat healthy, but whose work demands limit their time in the kitchen.

Royal Ice Cream Delight

This is for the person who is not talented in the kitchen or just received a phone call from a long-lost friend or worse yet, the boss and the person is going to be by in less than an hour. What are you going to do? You have to serve something. A whole meal is out, but few people turn down a dessert, and none will when they see what you have created. Best of all, no cooking is required, just a quick trip to the store and five minutes later you have a dessert that you can put in the freezer and pop out when the impromptu guests arrive. So get out your paper and pencil and get ready to run to the store.

1/2 gallon fat-free vanilla ice cream

1 package fat-free or reduced fat chocolate chip cookies Lite.

1 container fat free whipped topping

1 package frozen raspberries

1 container fat-free chocolate fudge topping or syrup

Thaw the package of frozen raspberries. Pour raspberries with juice into mixing bowl and set aside. Crumble cookies into about 3/4" square chunks and line the bottom of medium sized dessert bowls. Spoon a few berries and juice on top to the cookie chunks. Add a slice or scoop of ice cream. Top the ice cream with more cookie chunks and berries. Add another slice of ice cream topped with a few more berries and a scoop of the fat free whipped topping. Pour a teaspoon of raspberry juice over the topping followed by a tablespoon of chocolate fudge topping. Add a berry on the top for good measure and serve.

Nutrition Facts		each 3/4 cup serving contains	
Calories:	274.0	Sodium	146.0 mg
Total Fat:	2.4 g	Carbohydrate	69.8 g
Saturated Fat:	1.0 g	Dietary Fiber	2.0 g
Cholesterol:	0.0 mg	Protein	2.3 g

Stunning Apple Surprise

A stunning apple cobbler whose apple and cinnamon aroma will make your guests anxious for your dessert. With only 6 grams of fat per serving, this cobbler will be as good for you as it's aromas indicate.

The Apple Filling:

4 large apples	1/2 teaspoon cinnamon
1/3 cup sugar	1/4 teaspoon nutmeg
1 tablespoon cornstarch	1/3 cup orange juice

The Cobbler Topping:

1 cup all-purpose flour	1/2 cup fat free milk
1/2 cup sugar	1/4 cup low fat stick margarine
1-1/2 teaspoon baking powder	1/8 teaspoon salt

Preheat oven to 375F. Combine the sugar, cinnamon, cornstarch and nutmeg in a large mixing bowl and stir thoroughly. Add the orange juice and apples and again mix thoroughly. Coat a 11" x 7" baking dish with nonstick cooking spray. Distribute apples evenly across bottom of baking dish. In a medium sized mixing bowl combine the flour, baking powder, salt and most of the sugar. Keep a couple of spoon full's of sugar out to sprinkle on top of the cobbler topping. Stir in the margarine until the mixture is like coarse crumbs. Add the milk and stir only enough to moisten mixture. Spoon eight even mounds of topping onto the apple filling. Sprinkle topping with remaining sugar. Bake until a toothpick inserted in topping comes out clean, about 30 to 35 minutes. Serve warmly. Add a fat free whipped topping for excitement.

Makes 8 servings

Nutrition Facts		each serving contains	
Calories:	248.0	Sodium	176.0 mg
Total Fat:	5.9 g	Carbohydrate	48.8 g
Saturated Fat:	4.0 g	Dietary Fiber	3.2 g
Cholesterol:	15.8 mg	Protein	2.3 g

Lemon/Berry/Berry Frozen Delight

A frozen berry dessert that takes but minutes to prepare and has no fat. An amazing decadent dessert that is so easy to mix.

1/2 gallon lemon fat free sorbet
1 - 8 oz pack frozen raspberries
1 - 8 oz pack frozen strawberries
Fat free whipped topping
Maraschino cherries

Place frozen berries in a mixing bowl and mash into 1/2" to 3/4" sized chunks. Scoop in the sorbet and stir together slightly. Cover and freeze solid, about 3 hours, until ready to serve. Spoon combined sorbet and berries into bowls and top with fat free whipped topping and a stemmed maraschino cherry for decoration.

<u>Nutrition Facts</u>   <u>each 1/2 cup serving contains</u>

Calories:	128.0	Sodium	29.0 mg
Total Fat:	0.0 g	Carbohydrate	30.8 g
Saturated Fat:	0.0 g	Dietary Fiber	0.9 g
Cholesterol:	0.0 mg	Protein	1.3 g

Fresh Fruit Surprise

So easy to make and so stunning to look at, some will say it looks too good to eat, but a treat it is and so good for you.

3 apples, peeled, sliced and cored
3 peaches, peeled, sliced and cored
3 cups fresh raspberries
3 tablespoons honey
1 teaspoon lemon juice
1/8 teaspoon cinnamon

Puree all but a 1/2 cup of the raspberries in a blender. Strain and discard the seeds. If no blender, place all but 1/2 a cup of the raspberries in a sieve and with the back of a large spoon, mash the berries and force the juice through the sieve. Discard the seeds. Combine the honey, lemon juice and cinnamon with the raspberry juice. Set the 1/2 cup of whole fresh berries aside for garnish. Peel, slice and core 3 apples and 3 peaches into slender wedges. All this can be done in advance. Make sure to cover and refrigerate.

To serve: Spoon 2 tablespoons of raspberry sauce on a plate and alternately arrange the wedges slices of apple and peaches on the raspberry sauce. Drizzle the remaining raspberry juice over the wedges. Garnish with the remaining whole raspberries and serve.

Makes 6 servings

Nutrition Facts		each serving contains	
Calories:	144.0	Sodium	1.0 mg
Total Fat:	0.0 g	Carbohydrate	24.8 g
Saturated Fat:	0.0 g	Dietary Fiber	2.0 g
Cholesterol:	0.0 mg	Protein	1.3 g

Raspberry Supreme

Equally as good with strawberries, or blackberries or even blueberries.

4 cups of berries, crushed	1/2 cup orange juice
1/4 cup quick cooking tapioca	1/2 cup
Fat free whipped topping	Fat free ice cream cookies

Crush all but a few of the berries with the back of a large spoon in a sieve and discard the seeds. Keep a few berries out for garnish. In a 2-quart saucepan mix the raspberries, orange juice and tapioca. Let stand for 15 minutes. Stir in sugar. Bring to a boil and stir constantly until thickened, about 2 minutes. Remove from heat and cover and refrigerate.

To serve: Spoon into 4 dessert bowls, and top with fat free whipped topping and a whole berry or two with a fat free ice cream cookie on the side.

Makes about 4 servings

Nutrition Facts		each serving contains	
Calories:	204.0	Sodium	124.0 mg
Total Fat:	2.8 g	Carbohydrate	59.8 g
Saturated Fat:	0.4 g	Dietary Fiber	1.0 g
Cholesterol:	38.0 mg	Protein	6.3 g

Oh How Good Chocolate Shakes

A chocolate shake that has virtually no fat and is thick and creamy. A great addition to a barbecue. Combined with grilled veggie burgers, whole wheat buns and a low-fat potato salad and you will have a picnic that is healthy and good for you, the family and guest will also enjoy.

1 cup no fat vanilla ice cream
1/4 cup fat free milk
2 tablespoons chocolate syrup light
1 tablespoon malted milk powder

Combine all ingredients in a blender. No blender, use a portable mixer and blend until mixed in medium bowl.

Serve in a tall glass crowned with a dollop of fat free whipped topping.

Nutrition Facts   each 1 cup serving contains

Calories:	197.0	Sodium	165.0 mg
Total Fat:	1.0 g	Carbohydrate	38.8 g
Saturated Fat:	0.3 g	Dietary Fiber	0.0 g
Cholesterol:	2.0 mg	Protein	8.3 g

Apple/Pear Carmel Delight

Another easy to make dessert that has all the appearances of being the product of a culinary master yet is so simple to make but looks so special.

3 pears, peeled, sliced & cored

3 apples, peeled, sliced and cored.

5 cups water

1/2 cup sugar

1/2 cup fat-free caramel apple dip

1/2 cup orange juice

1 fresh lemon

4 cloves

cinnamon sticks

In an electric fry pan combine the water, orange juice, sugar, the juice from the lemon, cloves and 2 cinnamon sticks, stir thoroughly and then boil. Reduce heat to low simmer. Just above warm. Add the peeled, sliced and cored apples and pears. Simmer until tender, about 15 minutes. Turn off heat and let cool. In a microwave-safe bowl, heat the caramel dip 15 seconds, pause and stir. Heat another 30 seconds.

To serve: Scoop pears and apple slices from fry pan with serrated server and let drain. Alternate pear and apple slices in a circle on a dessert plate and drizzle with caramel sauce. Sprinkle with a pinch of ground clove. Garnish with a cinnamon stick.

Makes about 6 servings

<u>Nutrition Facts</u>   <u>each serving contains</u>

Calories:	175.0	Sodium	80.0 mg
Total Fat:	1.0 g	Carbohydrate	47.8 g
Saturated Fat:	0.1 g	Dietary Fiber	4.0 g
Cholesterol:	0.0 mg	Protein	1.3 g

Root Beer Tropical Float Surprise

A quick and simple dessert is a root beer float. It is a snap to prepare with a fat-free vanilla ice cream or chocolate ice cream or sorbet and a diet root beer. To add a hint of tropical excitement, add a quarter cup of pineapple juice.

2 scoops of fat free ice cream
1/4 cup pineapple juice
12 oz bottle diet root beer
Fat free whipped topping
Maraschino cherry for garnish

In a tall glass, pour in the pineapple juice and an iced-drink spoon of ice cream and stir until mixed. Add the 2 scoops of ice cream. Pour in the root beer. Stir with the tall drink spoon a couple of turns to blend the juice and root beer. Top with a dollop of whipped topping and a maraschino cherry.

Makes 1 serving

<u>Nutrition Facts</u>   <u>each serving contains</u>

Calories:	125.0	Sodium	70.0 mg
Total Fat:	0.0 g	Carbohydrate	27.0 g
Saturated Fat:	0.0 g	Dietary Fiber	0.0 g
Cholesterol:	0.0 mg	Protein	3.3 g

www.ingramcontent.com/pod-product-compliance
Lightning Source LLC
Chambersburg PA
CBHW051208120626
46547CB00013B/1258